S0-BXD-212

Cancer:
A New
Breakthrough

Cancer: A New Breakthrough

by

Virginia Wuerthele-Caspe Livingston, M.D.

Nash Publishing, Los Angeles

Library of Congress Catalog Card Number: 72-81848
Standard Book Number: 8402-1281-X

Published simultaneously in the United States and Canada
by Nash Publishing Corporation, 9255 Sunset Boulevard,
Los Angeles, California 90069.

Printed in the United States of America.

First Printing.

1741304

This book was written at the insistence of my dear husband
DR. AFTON MUNK LIVINGSTON
who abhors idleness, especially mine.

Dedicated with love to the memory of my father,
HERMAN WILLIAM WUERTHELE, M.D., F.A.C.P.
October 6, 1885 — January 5, 1967.
Hero of my childhood, inspiration of my youth,
friend and preceptor of my adult years.

Acknowledgment

For financial gifts I am indebted to: The Fleet Foundation of San Diego, The Kerr Foundation of New York, The Billy Casper Foundation of Chula Vista, Mr. Shelley Krasnow, Mrs. Agnes Gellert, Miss Lisa Gellert, innumerable friends, patients and well-wishers, and the University of San Diego for handling our financial affairs and providing laboratory space.

For assistance in preparation of this manuscript I wish to express appreciation to: Dr. Dean Burk, head of chemotherapy, National Institute of Health, Dr. H. B. Woodruff, Dr. Irene Corey Diller, Dr. Eleanor Alexander-Jackson, Miss Adelle Davis, Dr. Bernard Rimland, Dr. Curt W. Spanis, Mr. and Mrs. H. L. Scantlin, Mrs. Renate Streiter-Smith; Mrs. Gladys Towles Root for legal assistance; and Mr. and Mrs. Alexander Kassity, my mother and stepfather, for their encouragement during the writing of this book.

A special "thank you" to Mr. Joseph DeSilva for giving me the opportunity of presenting my work on his TV program "Open Forum," Channel 13, sponsored by the Retail Clerks Union, No. 770. His continuing encouragement and friendship are greatly appreciated not only by me but by his many friends and co workers. His compassion for his fellow men is exemplified by the many programs he has sponsored in the fields of nutrition, predictive medicine and public health.

Contents

Cancer:
A New
Breakthrough

Introduction

This dread disease reaches into every family around the world; it does not spare the nursing infant, the child, the teen-ager, the young adult, the busy mother, the providing father in his prime nor does it spare the old after many decades of useful life. One person dies of this disease in the United States every minute, 1400 a day and 350,000 a year. One person in four, 25 percent, will be stricken with it some time in the course of his lifetime. In the later decades of life, after fifty years of age, one person in three will be attacked. About 1,500,000 people are suffering with this disease at the present time. The total dead from the Vietnam War is 53,316, with 293,442 wounded. Motor vehicle accidents killed 54,800 and injured 2,000,000 in 1970. However, the vast majority of those injured in vehicular accidents will completely recover. The number who will be spared at least a year more after contracting the dread disease of cancer will be roughly one-third or less.

What is this hidden killer that destroys the just and the unjust, the young and the old, the famous and the humble, the rich and the poor, that strikes like a murderer in the dark to destroy the lives of millions of the inhabitants of the earth? The treasures of health and long life cannot be locked up in a safe. They cannot be hoarded for future use nor can they readily be bought or sold. This dread disease strikes as it will and when it will.

The common name for this epidemic disease is *cancer* meaning the *crab* because of its appearance in living tissue. It appears to have claws which spread among the body cells and reach out to entangle the surrounding structures in a relentless grip.

I have called the disease and the microbial agent we believe to be the causative agent the hidden killer — *Cryptocides*. During a meeting of the New York Academy of Sciences at the Waldorf-Astoria Hotel in New York in November 1969 were requested to classify the microorganism we were describing as the cause of cancer. All microorganisms are classified into groups according to their properties and given a name. This is called determinative bacteriology. The classification under a name is called nomenclature. All microorganisms are classified under an order, a family, a genus, a species, and variants.

The microorganism has been classified as follows:

Order: Actinomycetales
Family: Progenitoraceae
Genus: *Cryptocides*
Species: *Cryptocides tumefaciens;*
           Cryptocides sclerodermatis (Sclerobacillus)
               Wuerthele-Caspe, 1947;
           Cryptocides wilsonii, Wuerthele-Caspe,
               Alexander-Jackson, Diller, 1956.
Variants: hominis, rodentii, avii, etc.

Actinomycetales means that it is like the sun and has rays or armlike processes in its growth on being planted on cultural media which consists of selected biological material which acts

as the soil for the growth of organisms. It is called Progenitoraceae because it appears to be very primitive in its growth.
Forms resembling these organisms have been found in pre-
Cambrian rock long before man appeared upon the earth. Its
genus is *Cryptocides,* a combined Greek and Latin word which
means the hidden killer. Under species there are groups which
cause various diseases such as cancer, scleroderma (a hardening
of the skin) and other connective-tissue diseases. The variants
mean that it can occur in several different species such as man,
rodents and birds. The Actinomycetales also contain the microorganisms which cause tuberculosis and leprosy.

It is now commonly believed that cancer is an infectious
disease caused by a tumor agent described at times as a virus
and at other times as a C-particle because of its shape under the
microscope. The purpose of this book is to relate the disease of
cancer to an infectious agent, Progenitor *Cryptocides,* and to
describe how this hidden or occult infection produces the many
forms of the disease. Also, this book is intended to inform the
average person what he can do to protect himself by guarding
against this infection and what kinds of treatment may be
helpful once he has contracted the disease.

Thousands of dedicated people using millions of dollars the
world over are devoting their lives to the conquest of this
disease. Some are working in beautiful, well-funded and well-
equipped laboratories, with large amounts of money and material at their disposal. Others, equally qualified, but more
obscure, are working under great adversity with little money,
poor equipment and receive only discouragement from the
Establishment. Throughout history, not only in science and
medicine but in other fields, the man with the dream has
persisted in the face of every obstacle. It is human nature to
believe that what is acceptable today scientifically must be
enforced and perpetuated in our medical institutions. But the
average man rises up in rebellion against the dictates of established medical procedures. He asks, "Are you a cut, burn and
poison doctor?" Meanwhile the dreamer knows that tissue

destruction is not the answer, that there are other ways to utilize the wisdom of the human body, which, given assistance, can heal itself. The dreamer seeks to prevent and to heal using the protective mechanisms with which each of us is blessed. That dreamer may be a present-day Koch, Pasteur, or Semmelweiss. That day may be now.

The
Hidden Killer

An attractive woman and her husband entered our consultation room. Her beautiful clothes and careful make-up did not conceal the signs of her dreaded disease, cancer. Her moon-shaped face, under the make-up, had a waxy yellow pallor. Her cheeks and chin were covered with a thick, coarse fuzzy growth of hair. Her right arm was swollen tight against her sleeve and her right hand was puffy and blue in color. She was obviously wearing a wig. She had tied a soft white filmy scarf around her neck. As she sat down she crossed her ankles and placed her feet under the chair as far as she could, trying to conceal once shapely ankles now swollen and puffed over the top of her loose shoes. My husband and I, both physicians, knew before she spoke why she had come to see us.

Since our appearance in January and February 1972 on Joseph DeSilva's "Open Forum," Channel 13, Los Angeles, when we were interviewed on various aspects of cancer, our medical office in San Diego has been crowded with terminal cancer patients. This woman was one of the many who came seeking help. Her history was typical. As an intelligent person and a regular contributor to the American Cancer Society, she was aware of the seven signs of cancer. She had also seen the movie on self-examination of the breasts. So it was that three years ago, as was her monthly custom, halfway between her menstrual periods, she examined her breasts while lying down. At first she thought she was imagining things but after checking the left breast, which had some irregularities that were soft and rubbery, she knew that this lump was different. For three days she watched the lump. Since it did not change, she consulted her family physician. He sent her for a mammogram, an X-ray picture of the breast. This showed an area of density that strongly suggested a tumor mass. From there she was sent to a competent surgeon who scheduled her for breast surgery within the week. At the hospital she was thoroughly examined, with chest and skeletal X-rays as well as by a complete laboratory workup including blood typing. She signed an authorization for the surgeon to remove her breast and to perform a "radical mastectomy" if the frozen section of the small lump proved to be malignant. The surgeon explained that the lump would be removed and examined as a frozen specimen in the pathology laboratory by the pathologist while she was under anesthesia. If his verdict was "malignant" then, without returning to consciousness, she would have a radical mastectomy performed.

The tumor was malignant. The radical mastectomy was performed. Not only was the entire breast removed but the underlying muscles and all of the glands in the armpit as well.

The complete pathological report, made a few days later when she was able to walk around and was ready to be discharged from the hospital, stated that no nodes in the axilla, or armpit, were involved and that all of the tumor had been cut away. Her surgeon recommended, however, that she have both her ovaries removed because she was still having menstrual periods. He thought the breast cancer might be "estrogen dependent," that is, the hormones from the ovaries might have an effect on the possible residual tissues, causing new tumors to arise elsewhere in the body or in the scar from the removed breast. He advised a short rest period. She went home for two weeks then returned to the hospital and both ovaries were removed.

All went well in the hospital following the oophorectomy except that she began to have "hot flashes" due to the loss of estrogen, or female sex hormone, now that she no longer had her ovaries. She was told that she could never take estrogen and must learn to live with these symptoms. After the wound from the mastectomy healed and the stitches were removed, she was started on a series of cobalt treatments over the area of the surgery. She was advised that these were necessary to prevent the cancer from appearing in the scar and in the surrounding glands and tissues. This treatment meant a daily visit for four weeks to the hospital except for Sunday. She lost weight because of nausea and poor appetite. She was assured that she would feel much better when the cobalt series was completed.

After the radiation treatments she did feel much better. However, her right arm was quite swollen from the removal of the glands from the axilla. She then received physiotherapy treatments and was given exercises to return the arm to normal function. She went to a surgical supply firm and was fitted with an artificial breast, which helped her clothes to fit properly. The psychological trauma resulting from all of these procedures was tremendous, but she was fortunate in having a considerate husband who overlooked her depression and irritability, and teen-age children who remained loving and attentive. When she was sufficiently recovered, her husband took her on a European trip for several weeks. Gradually, she adjusted to the traumatic experience. She returned to her usual activities and rationalized that the whole situation was worthwhile because now she could look forward to a normal life.

A little more than a year later while drying herself after her usual morning shower, she suddenly felt some small pea-sized nodules along the old breast scar. All her former fears returned.

She hurried to her family physician who confirmed the fact that, indeed, there were several small lumps there but they were "just local" and could be taken care of with more X-ray treatment. Again she went to the radiologist who treated her with radiation. But even during the treatment fresh nodules appeared on both sides of her neck. More radiation was given. She was nauseous, weak and ill. Her skin became brawny, thick, purple in color, resembling the after-effects of a severe burn. Now she was told that male hormone treatment might help. She then received large doses of testosterone. Her voice deepened, her skin coarsened and pustular acne with a fuzzy growth of hair appeared on her cheeks and chin. She had some of the coarse black hairs removed with electrolysis. However, the nodules came back again. She was sent to a chemotherapist who prescribed 5 FU. As a result of this chemical treatment all of her hair fell out. She was assured that it would grow again. In the meantime she purchased a wig. However, before her hair began to regrow, she awoke one day to find that she could not bend over to put on her shoes. She had a sudden, excruciating pain in her back. The backs of both legs and thighs were very painful.

Again she consulted her family doctor. He returned her to the radiologist. He recommended that she have an X-ray scan of her skeleton, that is, X-ray pictures of the major bones of her body. She also had a chest X-ray. Her chest was clear but she had many bone lesions several of which were in the skull and some in the pelvis or bones of the hips and lower spine. This is what had caused the sudden back pain. She had difficulty in walking and developed a gait that resembled the waddle of a duck.

Her blood analysis now showed evidence of bone destruction and some liver impairment. Again she was advised that more chemotherapy or more hormone therapy could help her. By this time she was completely dispirited and lived without hope. She was taking pills frequently for pain. This went on for a number of months. There seemed to be some evidence of bone healing in a few areas but after several weeks the bone lesions progressed. Again she was advised to see her surgeon. After numerous consultations she was told that the removal of her adrenal glands could give her at least one year of remission with healing of her bones and soft tissue lesions.

These glands are situated just above the kidneys and perform an essential body function in producing the adrenal steroids that are necessary to life. It was explained that if the adrenals remained they could stimulate the remaining cancer lesions to further growth. In 25 to 50 percent of cases their removal could lead to a lessening of her symptoms for a year or possibly more. In some instances, a patient might even become free of symptoms for five or six years. However, she would be committed to taking steroid hormones by mouth or injection for the rest of her life in order to stay alive. Life had now become a series of horrendous experiences. She was numb with misery.

Again her loved ones and friends rallied around and told her that this time, surely, she would be helped. In a daze, she signed permission for the adrenalectomy. She was encouraged by the assurance that if this surgery was successful for a year or more, then at a later date, she could have her pituitary gland removed. This is a small gland at the base of the brain which regulates the other hormonal glands of the body. After its removal she would be required to take thyroid and pituitary extracts, in addition to the adrenal hormones, but she could gain a few more months or even a year or more by this last procedure. The adrenalectomy was performed.

Here she was, two months after the adrenalectomy, seated in our office. She had just finished giving her history. Her husband, his eyes filled with compassion, rested his right hand on her left arm, giving it gentle pressure from time to time as she told her wearisome and painful story. My husband and I, with averted eyes, tried to communicate concern, sympathy and deep interest by questioning her gently and quietly.

The nurse came to prepare her for examination in the examining room. As her husband started to follow her, she whispered to me, "Don't let him come in. Please ask him to wait outside."

We removed the covering sheet from her body. Experienced physicians that we are, we could only look at her with anguish and a sense of self-guilt that our profession had not rescued her from this dread disease but had mutilated her beyond recognition. The dark-rimmed beautiful eyes, the hairy, coarse, yellow face, the angry, furrowed deep red of the rhinoceros skin of her neck and chest, the nodules and ulcerations overlying the old mastectomy scar, the swollen abdomen with the wide transverse scars, the scars across her back, the thin swollen legs, the tremendously distorted right arm, the bent and shrunken body — was this once a lovely bride, a loving mother, a tender wife, a friend, a good neighbor, a woman concerned for her community, her country, her world? A spiritual being clothed in flesh?

As I placed my arm across her shoulders in an involuntary gesture of compassion, she whispered, "They said it would be better this time but I am no better; I am worse. There is no more help. I won't let my husband see me anymore nor sleep in the same room. I must spare him this agony. How much longer can I keep up? Doctor, shall I kill myself?"

This lady is only one of the many who daily come to our office seeking help. There is the man without a tongue who can swallow only in gulps, the woman wearing a tube fastened with tape across her face because she no longer has an esophagus, and is fed by a tube that leads directly into her stomach, the young blonde mother with her arm and shoulder amputated, the teen-age boy with his leg and half his pelvis removed, who sits outside in a car strumming his guitar while awaiting his turn.

The Search for the Hidden Killer

Because the microbe we named Progenitor *Cryptocides,* the ancestral or primordial hidden killer which we believe to be implicated in the cause of cancer, belongs to the Actinomycetales, it has certain properties that have been ascribed to other members of this group of microorganisms such as the tubercle and the lepra bacilli. These organisms, including the *Cryptocides,* are capable of retaining certain red dyes such as carbolfuchsin after decolorization with acid alcohol. This is a very important trait since it has permitted laboratory workers to differentiate between these organisms, which are pathogens, agents capable of causing disease, and other similar organisms such as colon bacilli, which are harmless and are present almost everywhere. This method was accidentally discovered by Robert Koch in 1882 after studying tuberculosis and enabled him to identify the tubercle bacillus as the cause of tuberculosis. When the acid-fast red-stained organisms are seen in sputum, it means that the person very likely has tuberculosis. The same method is applied to nasal smears and tissue preparations from people suspected of having leprosy, or Hansen's disease. In 1947 I found a strange, many-formed acid-fast organism present in all the cancers of man and animals studied. Until this time, although various kinds of cancer organisms had been seen and described by many workers, their universal property of acid-fastness was not known. I also noted that they are extremely variable in size and shape but always have some forms that are acid fast, which means that they can be identified and differentiated from other microbes that are not related to the cancer process.

The way the entire concept originated was as follows: I was the first woman to be a resident physician in New York City. At a dinner meeting where I met Dr. Jack Goldberg, Commissioner of Hospitals, I complained that a woman physician had never been appointed as a resident or chief intern in a hospital in New York. He promised to remedy the situation. In ten days I was called to his office where I was informed that I would be the resident in charge of the prison hospital for venereally infected prostitutes. This was not exactly what I had in mind when I asked for the appointment, but rather than refuse I accepted with the thought that the way would eventually be cleared for women to be residents in other fields. I found this one of the most rewarding experiences of my life. My preconceived notions of the prostitute underwent rapid reevaluation so that I developed a great compassion for these victims, often diseased and discarded by society. The prison hospital was behind a high wall in a compound that also included the infectious disease units of the city. I often made grand rounds with the other physicians and observed a great deal about several infectious diseases such as tuberculosis and leprosy.

Years later when I was a school physician in Newark, New Jersey, one of the school nurses asked me to help her. The nurse's condition was diagnosed as Raynaud's syndrome, a disease in which the ends of the fingers are ulcerated. The fingers appeared pinched and turned blue on mild exposure to cold. Also there were areas of hypersensitivity along the nerves of the arms and legs. On examining her, I found not only these signs but also a hole in the septum or dividing wall in the nose, a condition frequent in leprosy. There were not only hypersensitive areas of the skin but some that were hardly sensitive at all. In addition, there were patches of hardness. On reading about this disease, I decided that the nurse had Raynaud's disease as well as scleroderma. Scleroderma is a disorder resulting not only in hardening of the skin but involves all of the systems of the body with narrowing of the gastrointestinal tract, ulcerations, lung fibrosis and heart disease. It is frequently fatal in a few years if vital organs are affected. I thought it would not only be interesting but also helpful to make a study of this disease. I enlisted the cooperation of my medical friends, Dr. Eva Brodkin, a dermatologist, and Dr. Camille Mermod, a pathologist. We made smears from the nose and finger ulcers and stained them with the acid-fast dyes. To my gratified surprise, numerous organisms of the acid-fast type were demonstrable on the slides. We then obtained surgically aseptic subcutaneous specimens of affected lesions. Deep within the body tissue, as in leprosy, the minute red-dye-retaining microbes could be seen.

With Dr. Mermod's help, pure cultures of the organisms from human tissues were obtained and injected into experimental chicks and guinea pigs. I named the organism isolated from scleroderma, the *Sclerobacillus* Wuerthele-Caspe. The animals became diseased. Most of the chicks died, but the guinea pigs developed hard areas like scleroderma and in some cases, the areas appeared cancerous. The incidence of cancer in the guinea pig is only one in 500,000 so this occurrence was highly significant. Then I reasoned that perhaps scleroderma was a kind of slow cancer so I decided to examine cancer tissues by the same method using the acid-fast or Ziehl-Neelsen stain. In the meantime, with Dr. Brodkin and Dr. Mermod we published the original scleroderma papers concerning the *Sclerobacillus*. Del Motte and Van der Meiren in Brussels at the Pasteur Institute confirmed this work and reproduced scleroderma in the guinea pig in 1953. Years later, Alan Cantwell, a dermatologist of Kaiser-Permanente in Los Angeles independently found the same microorganism in scleroderma and related diseases. His work was published in the *Archives of Dermatology* in 1971.

On examining all kinds of cancer tissues obtained directly from the surgeon in the operating room to insure sterility and absolute freshness, I found that a similar microorganism was present in all of them. I enlisted the assistance of a well-known tissue sectionist, Dr. Roy M. Allen of Verona, New Jersey. This scientist prepared photographs of histological material for text-books describing cell structures. Using my preparations we were able to apply differential stains to the tissues and to demonstrate the presence of acid-fast microbes directly in the cancerous cells. I was delighted that the concept of the parasitization of the cancer cell by these organisms was verified. Also Dr. S.J. Rose of St. Michael's Hospital provided unlabeled material from which, in every case, I was able to pick out the cancerous from the healthy tissue by the presence or absence of the parasites. Both Dr. Allen and Dr. Rose joined me in the presentation of a paper in August 1948 before the New York Microscopical Society entitled, "Microorganisms Associated with Neoplasms."

From the beginning of the concept of the infectious nature of all cancers, I realized that the tumor agents described by such eminent men as Rous, Shope and Bittner, although classified at times as "viruses," would probably fall into this group of microorganisms since the *Cryptocides* have filterable or extremely small forms similar to viruses. The electron-microscope studies verified this concept. Photomicrographs in this earliest paper include also the demonstration of acid-fast organisms in all varieties of human cancers we have examined, as well as in Rous chicken sarcoma, and in coal-tar-induced cancer of the rabbit ear. Specific cultures were obtained on solid media used for the isolation of the tubercle bacillus. These cultures, however, appeared far more pleomorphic (they assumed a variety of sizes and shapes) than the tubercle bacillus on the same media. At this time through a mutual friend I learned of the work of Dr. Eleanor Alexander-Jackson of Cornell University. Dr. Jackson had succeeded in demonstrating that the tubercle bacillus undergoes many changes in morphology. She called these forms "zoogleals" which are today equivalent to the L-forms of Klieneberger-Nobel, the PPLO and the mycoplasms. These are intermediate forms of microorganisms which ordinarily have cell walls; but, in which, under certain circumstances the cell walls are absent. Some of these L-forms can be passed through very fine filters that hold back the usual bacteria and allow only very small particles such as viruses to pass through. In the past, the size of the filter opening or pore was used as a method to differentiate between bacterial forms and viruses but this method is no longer valid since we and others have proven that filter-passing bodies may regrow to become bacilli.

I was intrigued by the concept that bacteria are pleomorphic, that is, that they have a number of forms depending not only on the stage of their development, but also upon a number of other factors in their environment such as antibiotics and the presence of antibodies, substances made by man and animals which fight bacterial infection. Instead of a bacillus being a bacillus, *ad infinitum*, it can and does change into numerous other forms dictated by its need to survive or stimulated to greater productivity by an unusually favorable environment. Since man exists in a sea of microorganisms his ability to withstand them and their urge to survive often lead to a stage of symbiosis, that is, they live together. This can be on a competitive basis where the human keeps the bugs in check so that they are latent or resting. In some cases the captive microorganisms may play a useful role in producing certain vitamins for the host such as vitamin B-12. This is true of E. Coli a common inhabitant of the human bowel.

Dr. Eleanor Jackson and I then formed an association which continues to this time. She worked primarily with the tubercle and lepra bacillus in their various forms. Her work was largely restricted to the laboratory. I was a practicing physician with a strong bent toward medical research as my father, Dr. H.W.

Wuerthele, had been before me. I was to bring Eleanor concepts which she had never dreamed of and she was to provide me with the tools to establish the truth of these concepts. At the time, she was working in Dr. Wilson Smillie's laboratory at Cornell University. He was a stern curmudgeon not susceptible to new and foreign ideas. When we told him that we were growing an organism from scleroderma and that, very likely, there were similar organisms in other collagen diseases, he was about to toss Dr. Jackson and her strange friend out of his laboratory. However, one of the physicians at Cornell put us to the test by providing forty bloods of which a certain percentage were taken from patients with collagen diseases. With unerring accuracy we were able to demonstrate to him the twenty-two positive cases. Dr. Smillie became more sympathetic and tolerated us for the present.

During this period, the work of Dr. Irene Corey Diller of the Institute for Cancer Research in Philadelphia came to our attention because of an article in *Life* magazine. She was working with various infectious agents she had isolated from cancerous growths in animals. These agents were fungi and funguslike organisms, which often resemble the microbial forms with which we were working. We contacted her. She was most willing to cooperate with us. A lifetime friendship began and continues to the present with her and her husband, Dr. William Diller, Professor of Parasitology at the University of Pennsylvania.

When Eleanor and her father, Dr. Jerome Alexander, a noted colloid chemist, and her son Togwell were vacationing the following summer, I was struck with the thought that since cancer develops in the sclerodermic patches of the experimental animals inoculated with the pure scleroderma cultures, perhaps cancerous lesions have the same organisms. After working all summer, I greeted Eleanor with this news when she returned. She was horrified. She said, "For Pete's sake, don't tell Dr. Smillie. He's worried enough about you already. Perhaps it would be best that you stay away from the Cornell laboratory altogether. I want to finish my T.B. and leprosy work there where I have the facilities." I agreed to lay low on the cancer work and stay away from Cornell. However, Eleanor and her father continued to be very interested personally. Dr. Jerome Alexander generously contributed toward the cost of the page of colored illustrations in the first paper, "Microorganisms Associated with Neoplasms."

In the meantime, the scleroderma papers were well received. I equipped a laboratory in the basement of my home in Newark and proceeded with the cancer work alone. Eleanor Jackson, Irene and Bill Diller continued to advise and to collaborate at a distance. They came to visit whenever the opportunity arose.

How
the Work
on the
Hidden Killer
Started

My late husband, Dr. Joseph Caspe, a noted biochemist, and I were living in Newark, New Jersey, at the time of Pearl Harbor. Shortly thereafter he suffered a near-fatal coronary heart attack. At the time I was attending a few clinics and starting a small practice. We lost everything we had because he had invested his capital in a chemical business that required his full attention. However, he did survive the heart attack but was to be an invalid for several years until he made a gradual recovery. When we moved to Newark, a group of women physicians included me in their Journal Club. They were most friendly and congenial. When this tragedy struck us, Dr. Rose Bass, the head of the Journal Club called me and said that she knew we were in trouble. She offered to help us by getting me a medical job. Although she had a severe cardiac impairment herself due to old rheumatic heart disease, she hired a driver, called for me and drove me out to the Western Electric Plant in Kearny, New Jersey, which was close by. We had an appointment with the director. She recommended me highly and would not leave until I was told I could start the following week as an industrial doctor. Western Electric had 35,000 employees, mostly women, engaged in manufacturing communications equipment for World War II. It seems like yesterday when this thoughtful person, Rose Bass, took compassion on me and, unsolicited, threw me a life preserver in the form of a medical job.

I worked three and a half hours from 7:00 to 10:30 each morning at the plant. We examined applicants for jobs, appraised their physical defects, tested their eyesight, and hired them whenever possible. Grandmothers who had been rocking and knitting for years were hired just to tighten a single bolt on an assembly line. We had a saying then, "If they're warm, hire them." Sometimes we worked in the emergency room, which handled five hundred patients a day. Often we were obliged to work the late shift in order to take care of the night emergencies.

This job was not sufficient to meet our financial needs, so after the morning hours I hurried to the telephone company where I worked two more hours as an examining doctor, then I rushed to the Planned Parenthood Clinic and to the YWCA to do physical examinations or conduct counseling interviews. Later in the afternoon I returned home to do the marketing and to take care of my husband's needs. Evenings, my nurse from the Kearny plant came to help me in our apartment, where I had set up the guest room and the lobby as a medical office. There was an acute shortage of doctors. We often took care of the patients until eleven or twelve at night. I was happy that my husband was getting better. The varied medical experiences were interesting and my health was good, so I did not feel particularly tired or strained.

Some time before my husband's illness we had applied to adopt a child. In March 1943 our long-awaited baby girl was born and became ours through adoption. The night she was born I sat up drinking hot chocolate and nibbling on cold chicken (before I knew better) waiting for the phone call that would tell me whether we had a son or a daughter. The phone rang about three o'clock in the morning. I was so excited I swallowed a piece of chicken with a bone in it. I had to be hospitalized for three days and esophaguscoped to remove the chicken bone which was V-shaped and lodged with the points down in my esophagus. I looked weak and wan when we went on the first day of spring to bring home our child. She was six weeks premature and weighed less than four pounds but she was beautiful. My husband was thrilled to have a little one to care for during his convalescence. I arose at four o'clock in the morning to wash her diapers and to feed her the first meal of the day.

With time, my husband began to recover and was able to take some consultation jobs. We bought a big brick house on Mt. Prospect Avenue. The first floor became my office, the second floor our living quarters and the third floor we rented out. The basement later contained our laboratory. The house had twenty-two rooms and five bathrooms, and our little Julie had a fenced yard to play in. Suddenly World War II ended, Victory Day was upon us, and the Kearny plant laid off most of its employees, including me.

I needed a new job so I took the Civil Service examinations for school physician, made number one on the list and was immediately hired. I worked at the school in the morning and continued with the private practice I had now developed in the new house and office. I was doing everything as a general practitioner — delivering babies, assisting at surgery, making house calls, serving as director of a medical clinic for the indigent, delivering more babies at the Florence Crittenden Home for Unwed Mothers and working at the Planned Parenthood Clinic.

For our Julie we had a wonderful neighborhood grand-mother-nurse, Jenny Delaney, whom we called Laney. Julie and Laney frequently rode around in the car with me making house calls. Laney read stories and we sang. I often left them off in Branch Brook Park to play while I made hospital rounds.

Dr. Caspe was now well enough to take on the management of a factory in Patterson, New Jersey. It was at this time that I met Mrs. Grace Keeler, the nurse at the school where I was the physician. She was the lady who had Raynaud's disease with scleroderma. It was at her request I studied scleroderma, found the sclerobacillus and initiated the cancer work.

Shortly after this time I was appointed school physician for the Newark State Teachers' College which was quite an advantage as it paid better and was close to my home. Then I had more time to spend in my basement laboratory since I was no longer welcome at Cornell. Little Julie was my constant companion. When I went down to the basement to work, I told her that she could not come in because she might get sick from the things that were there.

I was using some of the Abbott Laboratory Products in the scleroderma work. Our scleroderma patients showed remarkable remission from scleroderma while under treatment. One of the company representatives said that the Abbott Company would like to make me a research grant but I would need a university affiliation. Due to state laws there were no medical schools in New Jersey. Rutgers University, situated at New Brunswick, had numerous branches around the state. Dr. Royal Schaaf, president of Newark Presbyterian Hospital said he would assign the old nurses' residence at the hospital to me for a laboratory if Rutgers would consider affiliation. I met with Dr. James Allison, director of the Bureau of Biological Research at Rutgers University. He was very much interested in the work I was doing and the confirmation by my associates. I found him most knowledgeable and cooperative. On June 2, 1949, I was officially made the head of the new Rutgers-Presbyterian Hospital Laboratory for the Study of Proliferative Diseases, Bureau of Biological research, Rutgers University.

When we were assigned the antiquated nurses' residence of the Presbyterian Hospital there were just three available rooms on the first floor which had previously been used for mailing and filing. It was a narrow, red-brick vertical building, with steep stone steps leading to the front door. It resembled one of the old brownstone Victorian houses of New York City. There was nothing very good about it except that it was rent-free and obviously better than working in a basement. There did not seem to be a great deal we could do with the Abbot grant of three thousand dollars and three small rooms in a dilapidated building. The people at Rutgers seemed to think that if we had a better building we could get additional research grants. None of the proposed grants, however, could be used for building construction and now that the hospital had given us the building, they felt that the rest was up to us. Meanwhile, the word had gotten around that we needed help.

A dynamic, attractive lady by the name of Nan Lupo, the wife of the owner of a moving van company, came to me with a proposal. It seems that she had heard of a miracle worker, a Welshman residing in London, who could cure cancer with plant extracts. His name was David Rees Evans. The story was that he had inherited a cancer remedy, consisting of an herbal preparation originated by his father and uncle in Cardigan, Wales, about 1905. It was based upon the healing powers of certain plants and roots of their native Welsh fields. It was reputed to have cured an older brother of cancer. Rees-Evans had been treating cancer patients in London since 1919. Mrs. Lupo visited his clinic in London and there witnessed great cures. Even members of the royal family had consulted him. (It might be noted that there is far less stringent control over nonqualified medical practitioners in England than in the United States.)

Mrs. Lupo came to make me a proposition. If I would agree to permit Rees Evans to treat a small number of cancer patients under my supervision, she would arrange to have all three floors of my dilapidated building completely renovated to my complete satisfaction. This was a very tempting proposal. I said I would present the idea to Dr. Royal Schaaf, president of the hospital, and to Dr. James Allison at Rutgers.

There were certain signed agreements I insisted upon:

1. Mrs. Lupo would procure the patients with their pathological diagnosis.

2. They would be referred by their own physicians.

3. I was in no way responsible for their treatment and an agreement was signed to that effect by each individual patient.

4. I would observe and evaluate their progress from time to time.

5. Their lives were not to be endangered, and they were to be referred back to their own physicians should any problem arise.

6. I would supply Rees Evans with a small number of mice implanted with standard tumors and controls for his use. I would have the mice autopsied and evaluated for tumor regression or suppression after treatment.

7. The work was to be conducted in secret; no publicity.

8. If the treatment proved to be successful, Rees-Evans was to consult a patent attorney and, with legal protection, divulge the ingredients of his treatment.

9. There was to be no release of any information until the hospital, the university, and I agreed to its release.

10. The above agreement was to be signed by all parties concerned.

Dr. Schaaf and Dr. Allison said that under these stipulations, we could permit Rees Evans to work in the small back room of the first floor of our laboratory. Mrs. Lupo wrote to Rees Evans and these regulations were agreed upon.

Mrs. Lupo was filled with a tremendous zeal. She felt that the world would now be saved from cancer since Rees Evans was to get his great opportunity to prove the infallibility of his herbal cancer cure. I was considerably less optimistic but was buoyed up by the prospects of the rehabilitation of the old building into a workable laboratory. Mr. and Mrs. Joseph Lupo were active in many of the Newark service clubs. Mrs. Lupo invited the heads of the various trade unions to see our building and to be honored at a luncheon. These good people came and pledged to remodel the building for us completely to meet our needs and to do so without remuneration. The broken glass in the windows was repaired, the rickety stairs reinforced, fresh linoleum was laid on all three floors, the dangerous wiring was replaced and high voltage wires put in for autoclaves and sterilizers, and the plumbing was replaced. Shelves and laboratory benches were built as were racks for animal cages. Refrigerators and a stove were donated. Usable chairs and desks were found. Even a hood with an exhaust pump was built to aid in sterile bacteriological procedures. The entire interior was painted and new Venetian blinds placed at the windows. I was deeply touched and grateful that these kind people came during their free time at night and on Sundays to give us such a gift of confidence and good will.

As a result of the rehabilitation of the building we applied for a number of substantial grants which we received and which financed our work for the following three years. These were from the American Cancer Society, the Damon Runyon Fund, the Rosenwald Foundation, the *Readers' Digest*, Charles Pfizer and Co., Lederle Laboratories, the Abbott Co., and many private individuals.

While we were staffing the laboratory and setting up our experimental program, Nan Lupo was preparing her home for the Rees Evans family. First David Rees Evans came, then his wife, then their son David, and then a daughter and various other Evans relatives and friends. Nan never lost her cheerful optimism. Untiringly, she drove Rees Evans back and forth to the laboratory, rounded up all the patients, helped me set up their records in a separate filing cabinet, and put herself and her resources completely at the command of the Rees Evans family. I could only be impressed by her dogged determination that Rees Evans have the opportunity to prove his claims. I fulfilled my part of the bargain by observing the patients and keeping careful notes on their progress.

Rees Evans' methods were as follows: he brought in small amounts of liquid materials which he applied to the skin over the lesions. While painting the skin of the patients he had little to communicate except that after a black mass formed and fell off that they would be "right as rain again." I watched a large black crust, or eschar, form over an inoperable cancer of the breast. The mass shriveled up and after two to three weeks it fell off. The skin seemed to heal. The breast was smaller but still quite hard. The patient was to die several months later of generalized systemic cancer.

Another patient, a man, with an inoperable sarcoma of the neck on whom the painting was done, died rather suddenly of a hemorrhage into the neck. A superficial skin cancer on an elderly lady's face fell off and healed. Cancer recurrences along the scar of an old breast surgery also healed.

The laboratory animals in no way favorably responded to the treatment since forming a black eschar on them was impossible and the material apparently could not be injected. Then I reported to Dr. Schaaf and to Mrs. Lupo that I felt that there might be some merit in superficial cancer of the skin particularly of the recurrent lesions on the chest wall after surgery, but I felt that the treatment had no dependable, predictable or discernible systemic effect. I reassured her that even this amount of success might be of value if larger numbers of such cases could be treated and the results compared with other methods of treating superficial cancer.

It was then the Fourth of July. We closed the laboratory for the day. On July 5th, when I returned to the laboratory, all of the file drawers were pulled out and rifled. All of the patients' confidential records with letters addressed to me from the referring physicians were gone. When I called Mrs. Lupo for an explanation she said that the reporter and the photographer from the *Picture Post*, similar to our *Life* magazine, had come from London. They waited until I was away for a full day to rifle the files and to take pictures of the patients. The Rees-Evans article appeared in the *Picture Post* September 9, 1950, in

England. It made great claims of success. Then began a great many transatlantic telephone calls from Sir Aneurin Bevan, British Minister of Health. When I consulted Dr. Schaaf and Dr. Allison as to our answer they advised me to handle the situation myself. I then cabled the English group as follows: "Work entirely experimental. No definitive results obtained. Rees Evans statements unwarranted and unauthorized. No results to be published. Would disavow all unproved claims by Rees Evans."

Nan Lupo left for a vacation. I never could censure her although she failed in the agreements we had made. She had consented to the rifling of the records and, in spite of the evidence, still felt that Rees Evans might have something of value to give to the world. Their poultice material might be of some value in the troublesome recurrent cancers along surgical scars and in difficult areas of skin cancer such as the lid margins of the eyes, but they put their own interest first. We learned later that the British Medical Society limited the Rees-Evans treatment to skin. We felt that, after all, perhaps we had served the English public to some extent.

As a result of this experience, I felt a real sympathy with Richard Guy, a member of the corporation of surgeons of London who founded Guy's Hospital, that ancient and gray stone building still in service in modern London. In 1759 Mr. Guy had published "An Essay on Scirrhous Tumours and Cancers, to which are added the Histories of Cases Cured by the Author by Means of Mr. Plunckett's Medicine." The Plunckett poultice had been a family secret for more than a century. Apparently, Mr. Guy obtined the formula and claimed to have treated a number of patients successfully without surgery. Since he did not divulge the formula he was assailed by his competitors. A study of cancer feuds over the centuries will show every feature of the quarrel of more than two centuries ago to be almost standard as a pattern of controversy over proposed but secret cancer cures.

However, I feel with complete conviction that whatever

"cures" may be proposed it is the duty and the responsibility of the proposer to make known his treatment and methods no matter what monetary loss he may suffer.

The Rutgers Laboratory in Newark

Now that we had the necessary facilities through the good offices of Rutgers University, we received many grants enabling us to expand. I became associate professor in the Bureau of Biological Research. In the meantime while Dr. Eleanor Jackson continued on her Rosenwald grant at Cornell, she decided to look into this cancer infection for herself. She obtained fresh tumors under sterile conditions from Memorial Hospital, which was associated with Cornell. After studying the cultures from these, she confirmed the fact that the specific organisms, the hidden killer, were present in all the tumors she examined. Eleanor left Cornell and commuted daily from New York to join us. We could now afford salaries for everyone. Dr. Eleanor Jackson was our bacteriologist; Dr. Roy Allen our histologist with a young woman to assist him in preparing tissue sections of our material; Dr. Lawrence W. Smith, our pathologist; Mr. Joseph Patti, an experienced animal-tumor expert from Memorial Center in New York; Marilyn Clark, a tissue culturist;

Andrew Steciuw, a Hungarian refugee who took excellent care of the experimental animals. We also had access to fresh cancer material from the hospital operating rooms. I was assigned a number of hospital beds to which I could bring cancer patients for study. We had the full cooperation of the Presbyterian Hospital under Dr. Royal Schaaf and of Rutgers University under Dr. James Allison. In those five years from 1949 to 1953 a great deal was accomplished.

We collected and studied all the obtainable animal tumors believed to be infectious in nature and supposedly caused by a virus. They were Rous, Walker, Sprague-Dawley, Shope, Sarcoma 180 and various types of fowl leukosis. From these we made cultures, bacterial isolates, which we compared with the cultures derived from many types of fresh uncontaminated human tumors, from blood, and other body fluids of patients who had advanced cancer. As anticipated, these cultures had a great similarity one to another. There were some variations as to size and some differences in the kind of media or material in which they would grow. Certain strains fermented one kind of sugar, some others. Some could live with little or no oxygen, some required more. Dr. Jackson studied various peptones or protein fractions until she found those that were best to produce good growth of the organisms in test tubes. I worked with making a medium from chick embryos. All of these supported the growth of the organisms very well. The organisms, later called Progenitor *Cryptocides*, were acid-fast and highly pleomorphic in their growth pattern. That is, they stained with the Ziehl-Neelsen stain in the same way as did the tubercle bacillus, which causes tuberculosis. This helped to classify them under the Actinomycetales. The bacteriologists at Rutgers University were satisfied that we had pure cultures free of contamination from other bacteria. Contamination is always the most important problem in the isolation of microorganisms. The contaminants are like weeds growing up in a rose garden. They are present everywhere. Usually they are harmless bacteria from the air or soil, or from humans or animals, but they may simulate the real culprits, the pathogens, the disease producers. No laboratory is ever free of them. Actually, it was the contamination of Sir Alexander Fleming's cultures by the penicillium mold that led to his famous discovery of penicillin that has saved untold lives. However, before starting animal inoculation, it is absolutely essentail that the cultures be pure and contain only one growth. Some of Jonas Salk's experiments on the immunity of monkeys were invalidated because one of the laboratory assistants anesthetized the monkeys using a mask that had not been sterilized. The mask carried the tubercle bacillus to the experimental animals and so most of them were infected. The experiments were completed before the break in technique was identified.

Our cultures were scrutinized over and over again. Strains were sent to many laboratories for identification. None could really classify them. They were something unknown. They had many forms but they always grew up again to be the same thing no matter how often they were cultured. They resembled the mycobacteria more than anything else. The tubercle bacillus is a mycobacterium or fungoid bacillus. Our advisors at Rutgers felt that we had pure, uncontaminated cultures and we were ready to prove Koch's law or postulates. Koch's law is the foolproof method of proving the cause of a disease. It is as follows:

1. The microorganism must be present in every case of the disease.

2. It must be possible to cultivate the microorganism outside the host in some artificial media.

3. The inoculation of this culture must produce the disease in a susceptible animal.

4. The microorganism must then be reobtained from these inoculated animals and cultured again.

We were able to fulfill Koch's law. The culmination of this work was published in the *American Journal of the Medical*

Sciences in December 1950. It was entitled "Cultural Properties and Pathogenicity of Certain Microorganisms Obtained from Various Proliferative and Neoplastic Diseases." There were six authors. In addition to myself and Dr. Jackson, there were Dr. John A. Anderson, head of the Department of Bacteriology at Rutgers, Dr. James Hillier, developer of the electron microscope and head of electron microscopy at the RCA Victor Laboratories in Princeton, New Jersey, Dr. Roy Allen, noted histologist, and Dr. Lawrence W. Smith, author of a well-known pathology textbook used in medical colleges.

This paper was the culmination of several years of effort starting with the scleroderma work. It required three months of scrutiny by the Rutgers group headed by Dr. James Allison and Dr. John Anderson berfore it passed their rigid requirements for publication. It stands as a milestone on the infectious nature of cancer caused by a tuberculosis-like microorganism, later classified as Progenitor *Cryptocides*, which has many forms in its growth pattern ranging from rather large mycelia to submicroscopic, viruslike particles that can be seen only with the electron microscope.

The pure cultures were obtained repeatedly from the various proliferative and neoplastic diseases of both men and animals. Then they were injected into animals capable of being infected. Gradually diseased areas developed which resembled those from which the cultures were obtained. Then the pure cultures were reisolated from the infected animals. Thus Koch's postulates were fulfilled to the satisfaction of the entire group.

It was our endeavor to show that the cancerous growth itself is not the whole disease. For more than one hundred years people like Rudolf Virchow thought the cancer cells themselves were parasites within the body. He did not understand that the small coccuslike granules he saw dividing in the cancers were not the development of daughter cells within mother cells but that rather, they represented the true intracellular parasite that was the causative agent. Recently in his book *The Savage Cell*, Patrick McGrady defines cancer as "A savage cell which somehow evades the laws of the body, corrupts the forces which normally protect the body, invades the well-ordered society of cells that surround it, colonizes distant areas, and as a finale to its cannibalistic orgy of flesh consuming flesh, commits suicide by destroying its host." This is a picturesque and dramatic description of the cancer cell but it is, fortunately, not entirely true. The whole truth may be that the parasite within the cancer transforms the normal cell into a sick cell that cannot mature by differentiation.

No one today believes that the initial chancre of syphilis or the late rubbery lesion called a gumma, which can appear anywhere in the body of an untreated person with syphilis, is the disease itself. Volumes have been written about the cause and cure of syphilis. The effects of the disease, like cancer, have reached into every corner of the civilized world. Mighty kings fathered syphilitic weaklings. The stigma bridging the generations became the basis for a famous play, *Ghosts*, by Ibsen. Then Fritz Schaudinn found the cause, the spirochete, Treponema *Pallidum*. The search for the cure began: injections of arsenicals, mercury, bismuth, to name but a few. These were often dangerous and not always effective. Such treatment gave rise to the famous saying, "One night with Venus and ten years with Mercury." Then came Fleming's great discovery. Now we can say *syphilis: penicillin*. All is said in two words.

Dr. Francisco Duran-Reynals in the years from 1940 to 1956 showed that Rous "virus" or tumor agent could cause acute and lethal hemorrhagic disease but latently, and by slow growth, cancer. With a still further repression of the tumor infectious agent, chronic, interstitial disease similar to arthritis and heart disease would appear in the experimental animals. He also proved that the Rous "virus" or tumor agent can cross species barriers and infect ducks and turkeys, and that filtrates, that is, filtered material from tumor tissue, not the cells themselves, can transmit Rous sarcoma to guinea pigs, rabbits, and marmosets.

Our classical paper, "Cultural Properties and Pathogenicity of Certain Microorganisms Obtained from Various Proliferative and Neoplastic Diseases," concerns not the transplantation of tumor cells nor even the use of filtrates, but the actual cultures made from the tumors. In other words, the living micro-organisms themselves, the Progenitor *Cryptocides*, the causative agent, were used in the animal experiments. It is the Progenitor *Cryptocides* that caused the disease in the animals and so fulfilled Koch's postulates or law. In 1948, I was years ahead of my time in showing that the Rous tumor agent was not a virus but a pleomorphic bacterium. As in Duran-Reynals's work, the tumors were only a part of the resultant disease. In addition to tumors, there were cheesy lesions or areas resembling tuber-culosis, which could invade any one of the essential organs such as the liver, kidney, heart or lung. These organs might show changes in the connective tissue, called collagen, which could lead to degeneration as seen in the chronic human degenerative diseases. So it was concluded that these microorganisms, P. *Cryptocides*, could not only cause cancer but a number of other ailments that afflict man. The infectious nature of arthri-tis, of some kinds of heart, liver and kidney impairment, and most recently of diabetes, has been proposed. Many medical researchers admit that the patterns of these diseases point to their latent infectious nature but none has come forth with the "antigen" or actual causative agent. It is these filterable forms that have been described as C-particles, mycoplasma or viruses by other research workers. We have proposed that certain strains of this Progenitor group may be the culprits.

Before the theory could be proven that the filterable form of the Progenitor group was equivalent to the so-called "tumor-viruse," it was necessary for us to spend many months with Dr. James Hillier of the RCA Victor Laboratories in Princeton. We passed the bacterial cultures isolated from the tumors of man and animals through filters that would permit passage only of so-called true viruses. These filtrates contained minute forms of life which then regrew to become bacterial cultures. This work proved conclusively that the Rous agent was not a virus. Peyton Rous did not call his tumor filtrates viruses but instead "tumor agents." His material could be dried and held on a shelf at room temperature for months and then, mixed with saline, it could be reactivated to initiate fresh tumors. A true virus has been defined as a submicroscopic infectious unit that lives only in the presence of living cells and cannot exist even momentarily outside of them. A great deal of time and effort has been spent in trying to find a virus implicated in any form of human cancer. *None has been found.* However, I propose that the filterable forms of P. *Cryptocides* which are of virus size are the causative agents in human and animal cancers.

The cancer organisms appear to resemble mycoplasma, organisms that exist without cell walls, expecially since the cytosine-guanine ratio of their nucleic acid, DNA, is similar to that of the mycoplasma. However, the usual mycoplasmas tend to remain in their state of existence without cell walls but the *Cryptocides* may pass rapidly through the stage without walls to the form of true bacteria and thus alter their C/G ratio. Perhaps all mycoplasma could be induced to become bacteria but this is still a disputed point.

Recently the consensus of opinion has been that true mycoplasma may not play a role in the causation of cancer. Dr. Robert Huebner, head of the National Institute of Allergy and Infectious Diseases, Bethesda, Maryland, believes that cancer is an infection. Of the various agents suspected, he feels that the C-particle is the most likely agent. It has been called by this name because the round bodies found in cancerous tissues often appear in a C shape. However, the comparison of the C-particles in mouse leukemia with the filtered *Cryptocides* isolates examined under the electron microscope show them to be similar in size and shape. In preparations from cultures the round forms are often seen to split and assume the C form. It would seem that this splitting into a C is characteristic, but not necessarily a method of identification. All the other methods are necessary as well.

There was some criticism that mice often had cancer spontaneously and that it would be better to try another animal.

However, in all research the results are judged by the comparison of the treated animal with the untreated controls so that even if there are cancers in the untreated, there is a significant differential. The need for genetically controlled mice led to the development of certain inbred strains that had predictable sites and numbers of tumors. We also used these strains. In addition we used guinea pigs. These animals are resistant to cancer having a natural immunity so that spontaneously only 1 in 50,000 develops cancer. We were able to produce tumors in 25 percent.

It was while working with guinea pigs that my suspicions as to the method of transmissibility of tumors were confirmed. Due to an error, the infected guinea pigs were housed in cages at the top of the racks while the healthy uninoculated controls, instead of being housed on different racks, were placed in cages underneath. To our surprise, the control animals also showed cancer. On careful inspection, we found that the droppings at times from the top cages fell into the drinking water and food of the guinea pigs below. From that time forward, we kept the controls in entirely separate rooms. Our animal man changed his gown, cap, mask and gloves in going from one area to the other. The guinea pig controls thereafter were negative.

We tried the effect of the cancer cultures on living tissue cultures. Tissue cultures consist of living cells grown in culture tubes. They are nourished by various types of nutritive material, some artificial and some from serum of chickens and calves. We found that under the influence of the microbes the tissue cultures showed marked changes such as degeneration and destruction with heavy doses, piling up of cells with smaller doses, vesiculation of some cells, and the appearance of abnormal mitoses in others. Abnormal mitoses indicate a cancerlike change because the cells do not divide normally. However, I suspected that the embryo fluids used for maintenance of the tissue cultures could contain the cancer agent since it came from chicks. This proved to be the case. Thereafter, whenever "spontaneous" conversion of a tissue culture to the cancerous state was described in the literature, I would be most skeptical as to the cause. Again it was the differential between the infected and uninfected tissue cultures that was significant in short-term studies. Later, the doctors Diller were to perform some excellent experiments with their cancer cultures in living tissue. They confirmed the conversion of normal cells to abnormal cells by the inoculation of the cancer microbes.

In "Intracellular Acid-fast Organisms Isolated from Malignant Tissues," page 143, the Dillers state that in tissue cultures, "it is possible that the spindle mechanism (the division process, which is disturbed in the cancer cell) was affected since there were abortive mitoses, as demonstrated by pairs of nuclei degenerating in the process of separation and by a high percentage of binucleates. At twenty-four hours the coccoid or small rod forms of the bacteria were closely applied to the cell surfaces as well as incorporated into the cytoplasm. The nucleoli also appeared to be infected. The fibroblasts as well as the epithelioid cells disappeared at the end of the experiment as a consequence of the presence of toxic products of cell degeneration and bacterial metabolism, and there remained only cellular debris and bacteria while control cultures were still flourishing."

We were constantly confronted with some problem or other, some serious and some humorous. We experimented with various types of tissues for our tissue cultures. I thought we should try some healthy young human cells. Happening to glance across the courtyard to the nurseries of the newborns in the hospital I thought to myself, "Now there's a wonderful source of healthy young human cells. I'll ask the doctor to save me the foreskins of the circumcized babies. I'll have them put in sterile gauze and immediately we'll bring them over to set them up in cultures. It's certainly worth a try."

So on an icy, cold, dark February morning, our tissue culturist, Marilyn Clark, went over to collect the morning's harvest of fresh foreskins. I glanced out of the window of the tissue culture room as Marilyn started across the icy courtyard carrying the neatly covered tray of foreskins. She was cold and she was hurrying. All of a sudden her feet flew out from under her and down she went, scooting along the ice. The tray flew out of her hands scattering foreskins into the air. Scarecely before they had a chance to reach the ground, a flock of sparrows hunched on a neighboring telephone wire, swooped down and in a twinkling, all the little pink and white delectable foreskins were snapped up much like the pink worms that appear on a grassy lawn after a summer shower. Marilyn got up, brushed herself off, picked up the tray and gathered up the gauze. When I saw that she was not hurt, I was convulsed with laughter. The thought that those cold, hungry little sparrows were unexpectedly treated to a delicious meal cheered me up for the rest of that gloomy day.

Sometimes the work that Dr. Jackson and I did was sad and unpleasant. It seemed to me that it was important to study one kind of human cancer thoroughly so we decided that the cancer of the human breast would be the most suitable since the cancers usually were enclosed within the breast and not subject to contamination from the bowel or adjoining structures. Also, they were a common type of cancer and not too hard to obtain. I collected thirty breasts that had been removed for cancer from the operating rooms. They were fresh from the surgeon's knife directly after the pathologist had obtained his specimens for sectioning. They were, of course, kept sterile. I brought them back to the laboratory where we dissected the cancers and the glands from under the arm, or axilla. We numbered the specimens, cultured not only the tumors but the glands as well, and compared them with the pathologists' reports. In all of the cases where we could obtain blood samples, we grew positive cultures from the blood. Also, even when the pathologist reported that the underarm glands were negative for tumor cells, the cancer organisms would develop from them when cultured. These results showed that cancer is not a localized but a generalized disease.

During the time we were at the Laboratory for Proliferative Diseases we had many interesting visitors. On one occasion Dr. George Clark, pathologist, from Scranton, Pennsylvania, came to see us. He reported on the successful culturing of Glover's cancer organism and development of metastasizing tumors in animals produced by cultures from human malignancy. We had never heard of Glover or his work before. What he called the "Glover organism" was undoubtedly the same organism with which we were working. For more than two hundred years the same organism has been discovered and rediscovered, named and renamed in practically every decade. Each discoverer added something to the knowledge about the cancer organism. I had discovered the fact that it is acid-fast, and associated it with other collagen diseases. We identified it as the so-called "cancer virus," and demonstrated its filterable stages by electron microscopy. Dr. Clark was an exceptionally well-trained pathologist and a member of the American College of Physicians. Most of Glover's work was unpublished. Dr. Clark and his associates had been invited to Washington to repeat the Glover work. Dr. Clark remained there for eight years under the supervision of Dr. George W. McCoy, Director of Public Health in Washington, D.C. The Washington bureau did not release the work so it had remained unpublished. At a later date in 1953 when our group was invited to present papers at the Sixth International Congress of Microbiology in Rome, I invited Dr. Clark to attend with us. He presented a scholarly paper. It was gratifying to me that after many sacrifices, tribulation and suppression of his work, I could give Dr. Clark the opportunity to publish it. Prior to the Rome meeting in March 1953, we all met in Scranton to compare notes with the earlier workers such as Dr. Jacob Engle, Dr. H. B. Leffler, and Dr. M. J. Scott. We also raised sufficient funds to bring Dr. Franz Gerlach from Germany to be honored in Scranton at a "Gerlach Day." He, too, had devoted much of his life in Vienna to the study of the cancer parasite which he called a "micromycete." It has always been my conviction that there is no place in research for jealousy or destructive competition. How often has a truth been suppressed or recognition been delayed because of selfish men who would not recognize the merit of a fellow worker.

While Dr. Clark was visiting us, he reported that Glover had been able to produce antibodies and antiserum in sheep and horses that were beneficial in the treatment of human cancer. Using Glover's method, we decided to try to reproduce his work by immunizing sheep with an attenuated or weakened culture. Dr. Harriette Vera, chief bacteriologist of the Baltimore Biological Laboratories, who had done much of the confirmatory work with our cultures, sent us a generous contribution which enabled us to perform this experiment. I had a patient in nearby Nutley who owned a dairy farm. He agreed to rent me a small pasture remote from his house and barns. Then I purchased a flock of twenty sheep and engaged a state veterinarian to assist us. He examined the sheep and found them free of disease. We attenuated some of the stock vaccines we had on hand such as cultures from human breast cancer, from a sarcoma of a young boy, from a human leukemia, from the Rous chicken tumor, from arthritis, and from fowl leukosis. We injected two sheep with each strain. After about four weeks the veterinarian reported that some of the sheep were getting sick. We went to see them at least weekly and provided him regularly with the attenuated vaccines from the cancer cultures which he used for immunization. Several ewes aborted their young. The fetuses were macerated. Some of the sheep developed very swollen painful joints and could scarcely graze. Others looked poorly and got thin. We realized that the vaccines which were attenuated were still alive and had not fully immunized the sheep but had diseased them. We asked the veterinarian to bleed the sheep in order to assay their serum for antibodies. We received the sterile sera but the sheep had to be destroyed and carried away for incineration. I was so concerned for fear the soil of the farmer's pasture might be contaminated that I sent for the Nutley fire department to burn over the entire field with all the fodder that had been given to the sheep. Nature would have to do the rest in sterilizing the soil.

Although the sheep had to be destroyed we learned a great

deal from that experiment. We learned that the fowl leukosis serum agglutinated in high dilution the cultures from the boy's sarcoma, that the breast cancer serum reacted with the human leukemia isolates, and that the Rous sarcoma serum reacted with all of the cultures. This meant that the cultures from the human cross-reacted with one another strongly and with the animal sera, showing that tumors are not tissue or species specific. This was a harrowing and costly experience so we decided not to attempt any more experiments with large animals.

We next turned our attention to fowl leukosis, a cancerous disease that was killing many fowl on the poultry farms of New Jersey. We went to Verona, New Jersey, to interview a chicken rancher we knew. He said that yes, indeed, he was losing about 25 percent of his chickens to fowl leukosis and that he didn't know what to do about it. We asked him if we might have some of his sick birds. He handed us three chickens which could no longer stand up. We took them to the laboratory and in a short time they were dead. We made cultures from their heart's blood. These grew to be the same kind of cultures as those derived from all of our other tumors.

We decided that this time we would completely inactivate the cultures. That is, we would be sure that they were killed before we used them to produce antibodies in rabbits. We ground up suspensions of the cancerous lesions and turned these into a tissue vaccine as well. Then we took the cultures that had grown from the tumors and passed them through many subcultures in test tubes to be sure that they were free of cells and turned them into a bacterial vaccine. We thoroughly immunized two sets of rabbits, one set with the tissue vaccine and the other one with the bacterial vaccine. We bled the rabbits and refrigerated the serum. Then we went back to the Verona rancher and asked him for six more dying chickens. All six chickens could no longer remain on their legs. Their heads fell over weakly, they lay on their sides twitching from time to time and their beaks were open. We placed two chickens into each group. Two we set aside died untreated before morning. Two we treated with the rabbit antiserum produced by tumor cell vaccine and two we treated with the rabbit antiserum from the bacterial vaccine. We then watched them carefully. In just a few hours all four got up on their legs and were able to drink water. We treated them for several days with all the rabbit serum we had. All four recovered completely. The ones that received the antitumor vaccine recovered more slowly and were somewhat stunted in growth. The two chickens treated with the bacterial vaccine antiserum became very vigorous, full-fleshed roosters. After several months we destroyed the stunted birds. They were found to be tumor-free. The other two roosters we kept for one year. One day while I was making rounds in the hospital, one of the patients remarked to me, "You'd think we were out in the country instead of in the middle of the city. Every morning at daylight a couple of roosters crow so loud we're all wakened out of a sound sleep. I wonder who's keeping them in the neighborhood?" I took the hint. When one of the janitors remarked that they were mighty fine looking birds and would make a nice dinner for someone, we gave them to him for his Christmas dinner. We knew that he could never find such beautiful birds anywhere on the market. The rabbit antiserum had cured the cancer in the chickens. Most important, it was the antiserum produced in the rabbits with the pure bacterial cultures that was the curative agent.

Association with other Research Groups

Although the research work we were doing was confirmed by many corroborative workers there continued to be considerable friction between our group and the groups that directed their efforts not toward the microbic cause of cancer but against the cancer cell itself. Their theory was that if you could destroy the cancer cell you could conquer the disease. This was the old theory that Rudolf Virchow had proposed so many years ago: that the cancer cell is parasitic upon the body and one has only to destroy it to conquer the disease. This is a completely erroneous principle persisting until the present day. How many patients have we seen over the years who have asked in complete bewilderment, "Doctor, why has my cancer come back? They said they got it all and now it is spread all over." The complete removal of the cancer may have some influence upon the course of the disease but it is not the determining factor in the survival of the patient. *Immunity is the answer.* If the patient is totally nonimmune the smallest cancer completely removed will not prevent many other cancers from arising in other parts of the body. Many of the large research centers, such as the Sloan-Kettering Memorial Hospital in New York City, near Cornell Medical School on 68th Street, under Dr. Cornelius P. Rhoads, were dedicated largely to finding a chemical or group of chemicals that would destroy the cancer cell. He would brook no competition or interference from any one who disagreed with his concepts. He considered us an upstart group. This included our collaborators as well. He was often heard to say, "When the cause and cure of cancer is found, I will find it." He died a disappointed man.

It is always amazing to me how the fallacious conclusions of a man or group of men, just because they are associated with a large institution that is heavily endowed, can sway the minds of scientists and physicians all over the world and blind them to the true facts. This was the case of Cornelius Rhoads. The Sloan-Kettering Hospital was heavily endowed with millions of dollars from private giants of industry. Rhoads wielded his authority as a heavy club. He himself was not really a scientist but rather was a promoter and a politician determined to prepetuate the powerful cancer interests vested in him and his institution. Actually Dr. Conrad Dobriner influenced much of his scientific thinking. Dr. Rhoads was committed to chemotherapy, and well he might be since he was head of chemical warfare during the Korean War. He tried to turn chemical warfare against the cancer cell within the human body. His great mistake was that he believed the cancer cell to be the causative agent of the disease and not the parasite contained within the cell. To unleash the horrors of chemical warfare and the atomic bomb in the form of a cobalt machine against the helpless victims of a microbic disease is illogical. He was not content to limit his theories to his own institution but was determined to dictate the research policies of the entire country. At one point he almost succeeded in destroying the basic biological and chemical work at the Institute for Cancer Research in Philadelphia and turning it into a conceptual satellite. Fortunately

Rhoads

he failed.

19 years

About 1950, Dr. Irene Diller of the Institute for Cancer Research in Philadelphia attempted to set up a symposium at the New York Academy of Sciences in New York in order to present a number of papers concerning our work on the microbic infectious nature of cancer. The meeting was killed by Dr. Rhoads. All he needed was something to discredit one of us. Dr. Diller had accepted the gift of several ultraviolet sterilizing lights for her laboratory from a commercial company. There were no strings attached. However, Dr. Rhoads used her acceptance of this gift to state that she had commercialized her work and therefore was not eligible to hold a symposium. It was to be 1969 before we finally had our symposium at the New York Academy of Sciences.

One day in 1951 Eleanor Jackson said to me, "I hate to bring this up but I have a lump in my left breast." She came over to my office where I examined her. She certainly did have a sizable hard mass in the inner upper quadrant of her left breast. There was no question in my mind as to what it was. She went to Dr. Frank Adair at the Memorial Center who arranged for her to have surgery. Before Christmas she had surgery. The tumor was malignant and she had a radical mastectomy. Dr. Jerome Alexander, her father, and I stood by anxiously during the surgery. While we were waiting my name was called over the loudspeaker to come to Dr. Rhoads's office. I went there immediately. He motioned me to a chair in his large luxurious office overlooking East 68th Street. He was an imposing, tall handsome man. He said to me, "You people can help us a great deal with our research." Many thoughts raced through my mind. I thought to myself that now Eleanor was herself afflicted with the disease, perhaps he had softened and would be more cooperative in our work. Then he continued, "We have been looking for a tumor such as she has. One on the inner side of the breast where the glands draining the tumor lie within the mediastinum. [This is an area between the lungs where the great vessels come from the heart. It is fairly inaccessible.] We would like to have someone to try out a new surgical technique. She could be the first one to have her sternum (that is the breast bone) split, permitting us to do a dissection around the heart and great vessels to remove the glands there. We have not been able to get permission from anyone for this surgery. She would be performing a great service in permitting us to do this as it would be an experiment to see how it would affect a patient and to determine the length of time she might survive." I was so shocked I was speechless. He was talking about my dear friend and loyal colleague and not an experimental animal. I was infuriated. I screamed at him "Not on your life. That is a cruel and disfiguring operation. Her body could be so shocked that she might not withstand the operation. She didn't even need a radical since her glands did not drain toward the axilla. I will oppose the idea with every ounce of persuasion I have." I left the room with tears in my eyes. He had not called me to his office to commiserate, to sympathize or to help but only to ask that Eleanor be sacrificed on his altar of research.

Eleanor came through the surgery splendidly. The next day when I told her what Dr. Rhoads wanted me to suggest to her, she was most idignant. "We should stand by what we believe. I won't have any cobalt or any further surgery. I'll watch my diet and take some vaccines." This she did. It is now twenty-two years since that fateful day. Eleanor says she has never had the slightest evidence of a return of her tumor. She recuperated rapidly and was back at the laboratory in a short time. Eleanor has always been a woman of great stamina and determination. Her daily trips to the Newark laboratory in the freezing cold or the blazing heat were feats of endurance worthy of an Olympic athlete. She left her apartment on Riverside Drive early in the morning, took the subway and then the Pennsylvania railroad to Newark, then a bus to the laboratory. It took at least one and a half hours. In really bad weather, she would take a cab from the Newark station. I drove her back to the station in the afternoon. She was always cheerful, eager, interested in our work. Every step of the way was a great adventure that we shared. Sometimes we differed and quarreled. Sometimes one of us thought we were put upon but then the light of reason would shine through and the offender would apologize. So this friendship has continued for twenty-five years. We are very different people but we have been held together in friendship all of these years by our interest in the microbial nature of cancer and each by faith in the integrity and good judgment of the other. My admiration for her father, Dr. Jerome Alexander, was profound. He was not only a brilliant chemist but a great humanitarian.

During the Newark years we made every effort to coordinate our work with related microbiological procedures. We visited a number of scientists who were interested in our approach to the cancer problem. In 1949 before Rutgers would consider accepting me and my projects under their auspices Dr. James Allison and I made a trip to Philadelphia to meet Dr. Margaret Lewis at the Wistar Institute. She and her husband had spent a lifetime of research in the microbiology of cancer, especially with the rat. She had stored paraffin blocks of experimental cancer in rats in her laboratory. After we had conversed for some time I said to her, "You can give me any one of those tumor blocks and I will demonstrate with proper staining the causative organisms in the sections." She was a delightful, helpful person so, at random, she took a block of tissue from the shelf. Even without the corroboration of the stained slides, she told Dr. Allison that she thought my work should be associated with Rutgers University. I turned the tissue block over to Dr. Roy Allen who prepared the sections with our special stains. Or course the "hidden killer" was revealed throughout the tumor by the acid-fast stain. We sent the stained sections to Dr. Lewis and to Dr. Allison.

After Dr. Eleanor Jackson joined our laboratory we made many trips to visit clinics and research centers. I was especially interested in meeting with Dr. Elise L'Esperance of the then Strang Memorial Cancer Detection Clinic at 444 East 68th Street,

New York City. Not only had she founded the first cancer detection clinic in the world but she had worked on the microbic theory of cancer. When I was a student at Bellevue Medical College, while studying pathology our professor said rather disparagingly, "There is a woman pathologist at Cornell who thinks Hodgkin's disease (a form of glandular cancer) is caused by avian tuberculosis. She has published a report on this but no one has confirmed her findings." As I looked into the microscope at the slides of Hodgkin's disease I could not help comparing them in my mind with the slides I had seen of tuberculosis. In Hodgkin's disease the large multinucleated giant cells are called Reed-Sternberg cells. They are similar to the giant cells of tuberculosis. In tuberculosis these cells form and engulf the tubercle bacilli. I stored away in my memory the thought that she was probably right but she would have a difficult time in gaining acceptance. After I had made my initial observations of the acid-fast tuberculosislike forms in scleroderma followed by my observations of the same forms in all cancers including Hodgkin's disease, I remembered Dr. L'Esperance.

About 1950, while we were at the Newark laboratory, I phoned Dr. L'Esperance. She said that she would be glad to see Eleanor and me. She asked us to meet her at the Strang Memorial Cancer Detection Clinic. I was most anxious to see the clinic. I knew something about the founding of the Strang center. Dr. L'Esperance was a pathologist. She had also been very active for years at the New York Women's Infirmary where she had also established a cancer detection center. She and her sister, Miss May Strang, were the nieces and heirs of Chauncey Depew, head of the New York Central Railroad and a famous after-dinner speaker. After his death the two women inherited a great deal of money. They founded the Kate Depew Strang Memorial Cancer Detection Clinic in memory of their mother who died of cancer. It was the first of its kind to be founded in the world.

We met with Dr. L'Esperance who greeted us cordially and

showed us around the clinic. In the first year the clinic was started, only forty-one patients went through. In the last eight months in 1950 from January to August more than two thousand were screened. During this time Dr. L'Esperance had established the validity and utility of the work of Dr. George N. Papanicolaou, M.D., Ph.D. Later he was called the Father of Modern Cytology because of his outstanding contributions in the field of exfoliative cytology. We met him that day in his laboratory. He was very pleasant and showed us some of his work. He is the reason why now the ladies are having their Pap smears regularly. The body cells that are cast off from the uterus, cervix and vagina are smeared from the cervix, are placed on a slide and stained. Not only is the presence of cancer cells detected but the amount of estrogen in the body is indicated by the size and shape of the nucleus of the cell in relation to the cytoplasm. This test is useful for determining the stage of menopause in women. Unfortunately, when the smear for cancer is positive, the cancer is already there. However, it does permit early detection of some kinds of cancer of the female reproductive organs. The same method of cell determination is now applied to a number of other sites such as lung and stomach. Until Dr. L'Esperance demonstrated the usefulness of the Pap smear at her cancer detection clinics, the work of Dr. Papanicolaou was not accepted.

It was a thrill for me to tell her that I had found acid-fast organisms that seemed to be similar to the ones she had observed in Hodgkin's disease in all tumors examined. I told her that we had cultured them and that they were producing tumors in experimental animals. She said she hoped that we would have better success than she had when she was doing her early work with Hodgkin's disease. She said she had isolated the acid-fast organisms from the glands of patients, made a culture and then inoculated them into guinea pigs. She reproduced the lesions and cultured the organisms out again, fulfilling Koch's postulates. When she showed the animal tissues to Dr. James Ewing, the great pathologist at the medical center, he confirmed the fact that the tissues were Hodgkin's disease. Then when she told him that they were from the experimentally inoculated guinea pigs he said that of course they were not Hodgkin's disease, that it was impossible to reproduce the disease by cultures. Dr. L'Esperance was disgusted but continued on with her work until the technician she depended upon became ill and she couldn't replace her. She said that she was much more interested now in preventive measures and in early detection.

Of all the cancer diseases, the early detection of breast cancer is most useful and can lead to marked prolongation of life. However, no method presently known makes it entirely predictable as to which patient will be saved. She told us that she was greatly interested in women in medicine and had done a great deal to assist them financially. I shall always remember Dr. Elise L'Esperance. She was a striking personality; she loved beautiful hats and had an inexhaustible supply of them made by Molly of New York. The day we met with her she was wearing a gorgeous plumed one that swept down over the shoulder of her white laboratory coat. She was tall and slender and had legs like a race horse. She always wore high heels. She was a most elegant and vivacious lady. She told us on parting that she was going to devote the rest of her life to her ponies. She loved to show her hackney ponies at horse shows. She retired to Pelham, New York, and did just that. The last time I saw her was on a televised horse show at Madison Square Garden. She was sitting tall on the seat of her gig with her high-stepping pony moving along at a fast clip. As always, she was elegant. She held the reins in a gloved hand. Her back was straight and her feet firmly planted. The plumes on her hat streamed grandly behind her over the sable fur stole draped casually around her shoulders. She died in 1958 of cancer of the liver. I hope I shall see that gallant lady again. Ironically, Dr. James Ewing died of cancer also. Her sister, Miss May Strang also died of the dread disease that Dr. L'Experance fought so devotedly to conquer.

During 1950 we made many trips to Princeton to take our filtered cultures to Dr. James Hillier of the RCA Victor Laboratories for electronmicroscopy. Dr. Hillier was very exacting in his studies of the microbe *Cryptocides*, the hidden killer. Many of the smaller bodies were beyond the range of the light microscope and were filterable on the basis of size alone. Repeated electron microscopic studies were made before and after passage through mice of pure microbic strains isolated from patients with cancer and with scleroderma, and from chickens infected with the Rous "virus" or tumor agent. The filtered bodies appeared to be the same size as "viruses." An electron photograph of the particles seen in mouse leukemia and a similar one of the microbic structures we isolated in culture illustrated the fact that the bodies in the mouse tissues and those we cultured are undoubtedly the same agent. We feel that these studies definitely demonstrate that the so-called "virus," or the C-particles, or the L-forms or whatever name they are currently described by which we have often demonstrated in cancers of all kinds are the filterable forms of this microbe, the hidden killer, the *Cryptocides*. We exhibited our electron work at a number of meetings and received great commendation and an award of merit on one occasion. These cancer microbes are so tough and resistant to heat that at our 1953 exhibit at the New York American Medical Association Exhibit, the microbes stayed alive for five days while being televised by closed circuitry on a large screen hanging from the ceiling. The visitors could see the live bugs swimming about through the microscope on television. We were the sensation of the exhibit. We were indebted to the RCA Victor people for providing the television setup and an engineer to operate it for an entire week. The press coverage would have been great but again Dr. Rhoads forebade the publicity people to interview us. They were intimidated and did not mention our exhibit at all although we had crowds of people waiting to get into our booth.

We had many other meetings of great interest. We visited Dr. Peyton Rous at the Rockefeller Institute. He was very kindly and interested in our work. We told him about growing the

Rous agent in artificial media outside of the living cell. He said that he did not think this was unlikely or impossible. When he received the Nobel prize in medicine in 1966 at the age of 87, it was more than a half century since he had reported the infectious nature of the first chicken tumor which later bore his name. We met with Dr. Richard Shope, also of the Rockefeller Institute, who had identified the infectious agent of a rabbit tumor. On one occasion at a meeting in Newark I had the temerity to differ with Dr. Shope on the type of cell in the Rous tumor which would transmit the cancer. He claimed that only the tumor cell could infect fresh chickens. I insisted that this was not true, that any cell of the infected chicken could pass on the cancer, that it need not be a cancer cell but any seemingly normal cell from the infected host could do so. In the case of blood, the serum had to be washed away but the red blood cell itself could transmit the disease as well as any other cell whether cancerous or not. To me this was and is an extremely important point because whether a chicken displays a cancerous growth or not, it may still contain the cancerous infectious agent within its body thus justifying the name of the hidden killer. This is the reason that it is not advisable for the cancer patient to eat poultry or eggs since it is impossible even by direct examination to determine which egg or which chicken is carrying the latent infection. Since it is transmissible to the ape, it is obvious that it can be transmitted to a susceptible human. However, Dr. Shope took issue with me and did not agree but he promised to look up the information. In a few days a letter of apology arrived stating that my premise was correct and that he had been misinformed. He was a generous enough man to acknowledge his mistake.

We also visited the Lederle Laboratories at Pearl River where we became acquainted with Mr. Paul Little who was in charge of their antitumor agent screening program. He worked largely with the Rous sarcoma. At this time Lederle was excited about the antifolic acid agents, the folic-acid antagonists. Folic acid, a B-vitamin, is the fraction from the liver that is essential for the revention of pernicious anemia, a form of anemia which formerly was fatal until the protective effect of liver and, later, folic acid was discovered. It is truly a life-saving food ingredient. At the time we were visiting Lederle Laboratories it was felt that substances that substituted for and opposed folic acid could destroy tumors. These are called analogues, counterfeits of the real vitamin made to fool the cancer cell in its requirement for the essential vitamin. The cancer incorporates the counterfeit into the cell and is killed. This is a kind of Trojan horse. Dr. Sidney Farber of Children's Hospital in Boston initiated the era of analogues in cancer in 1948. Some children show a remarkable return to health but the recovery is only temporary. At best a few live up to a year or more. This drug is called aminopterin and it is in use today. This minor success touched off a search for analogues, false vitamins, false hormones and other chemical agents. However, I was not impressed because chickens infected with Rous sarcoma virus, even though tumors did not develop, either died of folic-acid deprivation or other forms of the Rous disease. I warned Mr. Little that our bacterial cultures of the Rous-infected chickens treated with the folic-acid antagonists showed no diminution in the amount of growth of the causative agent. We had many round-table discussions at Lederle with the staff. Although conducted in a congenial atmosphere the conversations ended in a draw or stalemate. I couldn't agree with them and they thought a bacterial culture from a so-called "virus"-induced tumor, such as Rous sarcoma, is impossible.

On another occasion we went to the Bronx Botanical Gardens to request some cultures of *Bacterium tumefaciens*. Although Erwin Frink Smith discovered *Bacterium tumefaciens* in January 1908 he did not report his production of malignant growth in plants with this microorganism until April 1916 in the *Journal of Cancer Research*. He was a noted plant pathologist in charge of the laboratory of plant pathology for the U.S. Department of Agriculture. He was also a bacteriologist and president of the Society of American Bacteriologists in 1906.

He produced cancers in plants at will by injections of *Bacterium tumefaciens*. In plants these tumors are called crown galls and the diseased plants can be seen anywhere in the United States if one just looks for them. A number of investigators thought that *Bacterium tumefaciens* could produce cancers in animals and perhaps even in men. The work of Erwin F. Smith had a profound influence on Dr. Charles Mayo of the famed Mayo Clinic who reported on October 28, 1925, at an American College of Surgeons meeting:

"Down in Washington, in the government laboratories of the Department of Agriculture, Erwin Smith, a very well-known government bacteriologist, is carrying on a most interesting series of experiments on plants. He has rows on rows of plants in which he has been able to transplant cancer, resembling the disease in human beings. So exact are his experiments that he is able to foretell with absolute accuracy just how long it will require the cancerous growth to break out on the plant stock and more than that, just where it will break out."

We were given a tube of the living microbes and were admonished not to drop the bottle as we had enough there to infect half of the state of New York. Needless to say, Eleanor held the bottle very gingerly while I drove back to the Newark laboratory. We observed the microbes in culture and then injected a living culture into mice. With large doses the mice died overnight, with small doses they lived longer. Dr. Franz Gerlach was at the laboratory at the time and he thought that on gross examination the diseased tissues resembled sarcomas. However, we did not pursue this study any further except to make note that the culture was pathogenic for mice on injection. We have electron photographs of this culture. The organism appears to be endemic in the soil but it may also be transmitted by an insect vector. We had a young peach tree in our yard which appeared healthy and had pretty blossoms in spring. However, several of the peaches that ripened on it had tumorous swellings on them. On staining these tumors we found bacilli. I warned my husband not to eat the peaches but to cut down the tree and to burn it. I have always felt that all trees and vegetation bearing the crown gall should be destroyed by burning and the underlying soil sterilized if possible.

Of our many associations, our visits with doctors Irene and William Diller of Philadelphia were the most rewarding and enjoyable. Dr. Irene Diller, editor of the biological journal *Growth* is associated with the Institute for Cancer Research at Fox Chase, Philadelphia. She is not only a famous research scientist in the field of animal tumors but also a linguist, interpreter at scientific meetings, scientific librarian, cytologist, and authority on chemotherapeutic agents and their affects on tumorous and normal tissues of animals. She is especially interested in the relationship of microorganisms to cancerous tissues. Irene has always been a fount of information concerning research in other countries. She kept us abreast of much of the foreign literature. At the Scranton meeting in 1953 her paper was entitled, "Studies of Fungoidal Forms Found in Malignancy." She discussed fungoidal forms found as contaminants in animal tumors and other types of organisms which seem to have a more specific relationship to cancer. At that time Irene had not worked with the mycobacteriumlike microbe that we were later to designate as Progenitor *Cryptocides.* In later years, after she began to work with the same type of microbes that we were isolating, she did a monumental work in fulfilling Koch's postulates with her isolates by increasing production of tumors in mice of known spontaneous tumor incidence.

She also demonstrated by her blood-culture method that of fifty-six mice that became tumor-bearing during their lifetime, forty-nine or 93 percent were carrying the organism in their blood by one year of age. In 1,400 additional mice studied by this method, a very high correlation was established between the presence of the organisms in the blood and the eventual production of tumors.

She was often our severest critic but she maintained and

sustained our association with other scientists in the cancer field because of her wide acquaintance through her editorship of *Growth* and other worldwide contacts. Her work was, in general, confirmatory of ours and she made many additional contributions. She has an exactitude of technique that has eluded less scholarly investigators. Her statistical studies are not only convincing but conclusive.

When Dr. Diller placed well-known fungi such as baker's and brewer's yeast onto cancer cultures, the yeast killed the cancer cells. Sometimes the yeast cells killed the cancer cells without contact through secretion of some kind of antibioticlike substance. Injected into mice with transplanted tumors, the yeast destroyed the cancers completely in up to 95 percent of the animals. Two polysaccharides, zymosan and hydroglucan, were isolated from the yeast cells. They stimulated the reticuloendothelial system (RES) and cured some mouse cancers. The RES consists of cells that line the pockets or sinusoids of the liver and spleen and are present in bone marrow. The cells they produce act as guardians to engulf microbes and harmful materials that are present in the body.

The Newark Laboratory Closes

It was finally the long arm of Dr. Cornelius "Dusty" P. Rhoads that closed the Newark laboratory. On April 10, 1951, the *Newark Evening News* announced that $750,000 in cancer research funds were given to the Presbyterian Hospital in Newark. The same amount was given to the Memorial Center for Cancer in New York, which Dr. Rhoads headed. The trustees of the Black-Stevenson Cancer Foundation had sifted more than five thousand suggestions on how the funds should be distributed. In announcing the grants, the trustees, Charles R. Hardin, Newark lawyer, and Alfred S. Black expressed the hope that Presbyterian Hospital in years to come would develop into a leading cancer center. The foundation was set in the estates of two South Orange sisters. The accumulated residuary estate, of $1,500,000 was left in trust "for the charitable purpose of providing treatment and care both preventive and remedial, for needy persons who may be afflicted or threatened with the disease of cancer." The bequest stemmed from the tragic death from cancer of Mrs. Black's husband, John A. Black, in 1921 only two years after their marriage. It was also specified that the funds go to an institution in New Jersey or in New York. There was a five-year deadline for the disbursement of the funds. Mr. Black, the brother of the deceased, went to Billy Rose to make an appeal for help. The *Newark Evening News* published a column asking for suggestions.

More than five thousand replies were sent in. The trustees, after much deliberation, said that the Presbyterian and the Memorial hospitals best met the conditions of the estate. In discussing the gift to Presbyterian, Hardin and Black said that "although it is a general hospital as contrasted to the reputation of Memorial Center as the best-known cancer institution in the world, Presbyterian's personnel and associations are adaptable to a degree of specialization in the treatment and prevention of cancer. Presbyterian conducts a cancer clinic and a speech clinic for laryngectomized patients. Cooperative research activities on cancer supported by grants from the Damon Runyon Fund, Abbott Laboratories and the American Cancer Society are being conducted on the premises by the Presbyterian Branch of Rutgers University Bureau of Biological Research." Officials of the two hospitals then gave written agreements pledging faith with the vision of the two sisters for helping cancer victims.

We were not to know how that faith was betrayed for more than a year. As Mr. Hardin lay dying of cancer in the Memorial Center, he was prevailed upon to sign a codicil to the bequest stating that the Presbyterian Hospital could not expend its share of the grant without the permission of the Memorial Center. The only acquisition that Dr. Rhoads would grant was for a new wing to be added to the hospital and a high voltage cobalt machine to be installed. The sisters Black were betrayed as were Dr. Jackson and myself who had labored so long and diligently to establish a top-flight research laboratory devoted to the biological approach to the treatment of cancer. It was our work that brought the gift to Presbyterian yet it was this gift that destroyed all that we had accomplished.

At the time of the announcement of the Black grant, we were filled with elation. We could foresee establishment of preventive clinics which would screen patients and immunize them with vaccines when they were bacteriologically positive, clinics that would promote better life habits, better nutrition, safer and cleaner surroundings, industrial and environmental control of carcinogens, earlier detection of precancerous lesions and genetic counseling. It was a great dream while it lasted. We were not to know for some time that it was to be cruelly shattered.

In the meantime we were conducting our animal immunization programs, exhibiting at numerous medical and scientific meetings and preparing our material for presentation at the Sixth International Congress for Microbiology in Rome. After exhibiting at the American Medical Association Conference in June 1953, we left on August 5 for Europe. We all traveled together—Dr. Caspe, Julie and I, Dr. Jerome Alexander, Eleanor and Toggy, her son. We sailed first-class on the *Queen Elizabeth* on a torrid, oppressive day. Dr. Leo Szilard of atomic-bomb fame, had spent considerable time with us discussing our papers to be presented in Rome.

We could afford this expensive trip and the eight weeks in Europe without requesting any of the funds from our grants because Dr. Caspe, my late husband, had been commissioned and invited to come to London as a consultant to the British Fur and Leather Industry. He was an outstanding chemist not only in the field of biologicals and drugs but in the dye and tanning industries. His processes were known the world over. He had developed a method for straightening sheep wool into a flat, short silky fur by shearing and processing. He was able to dye these skins with soft, pastel colors for many articles of clothing. We had also bred mink and blue fox in captivity at our Blue Stock Ranch in Woodstock, New York. In the summer of 1953 Dr. Caspe was well recovered from the serious heart attack he had suffered ten years before.

We were received with much pomp and ceremony on our arrival in London. We stayed in London a total of three weeks.

Dr. Caspe spent his time visiting the fur factories and the tanneries with Dr. David Garrod, his English counterpart. Their company had just made a magnificent mink coat which was presented to Queen Elizabeth on the occasion of her coronation. Mostly Eleanor and I discussed our upcoming papers and the work of our colleagues who would be participating. We were particularly interested in meeting with Dr. Emmy Klieneberger-Nobel at the Lister Institute. She is the scientist who first described L-forms of bacteria. She called them L-forms for Lister Institute, where she was doing her research. The L-forms are bacterial forms without cell walls. They have also been described as bacteroids by some people in the United States and as pleuro-pneumonialike organisms (PPLO) and also as mycoplasma. In some cases these are basically the same. However, the mycoplasma appear to reproduce continuously under some conditions in the same stage, with the absence of cell walls, while the other forms have a tendency to revert more quickly to the more stable bacillary or coccal forms of origin.

We visited Dr. Klieneberger-Nobel at the Lister Institute, an old tremendous stone building with extremely high ceilings and large wide staircases. By our standards, the building and the equipment would be considered antiquated but the work that was done there was basic in microbiology, and served as pacemaker for years to come. The recognition of these L-forms and their relationship not only to the bacillary and fungal forms but to the filterable stages of the *Cryptocides* is most important. The L-forms are the link between bacteria and the viruslike minute bodies that are a stage in the life cycle of microorganisms. Many viruses may actually be L-forms of microbes which, under certain conditions, may be induced to return to their original forms. Previously the appearance of the adult and L-forms led to the erroneous conclusion that there was a mixture of microorganisms, a contamination of pure strains with other nonrelevant microorganisms. This erroneous misconception may persist today in examining isolates from cancerous material. Many bacteriologists are trained in the classical approach to the identification of bacteria according to standard textbook procedures. They see a coccus form and assume it is a staphylococcus or a rod that resembles a colon bacillus. Some true contaminants are readily recognized by their growth pattern but the *Cryptocides* is a great simulator of other organisms. It requires infinite patience to observe its growth pattern and to recognize its transition from one form into another. This is why the work of Klieneberger-Nobel is a milestone in microbiology.

While we were in London we spent a day with Dr. Ernest Brieger of the Strangeways Laboratory at Cambridge University. He had worked both in England and in the United States on the filterable forms of the tubercle bacillus by the use of electron microscopy. A number of previous investigators had described a complex life cycle for the tubercle bacillus, among them Leon Grigoraki. However, Grigoraki did not carry the work to the filter-passing stage nor did he have the electron microscope to demonstrate these forms that are invisible in the light microscope.

After Dr. Caspe completed his consultations, we flew from London to Frankfurt, the nearest air terminal, to Bad Kreuznach, where we planned to visit Dr. Wilhelm von Brehmer, who had worked with the same microorganism we have called *Cryptocides,* the hidden killer. Of course he had called it by another name, *Syphonospora Polymorpha* Von Brehmer.

The Inn Bad Kreuznach was delightful. It was on the bank of a swift-flowing stream. We reached the inn by walking over a wooden footbridge. There were beautiful tall trees and shrubbery surrounding the flower gardens and woodland paths. We kept the children at the inn, away from the town.

In the morning Dr. Alexander phoned Dr. Von Brehmer. In very short order Dr. Von Brehmer and four of his laboratory assistants arrived in time for a large German breakfast.

We were invited one afternoon to his laboratory in a small old house. We tried to learn something about his darkfield techniques with blood but did not succeed in observing any of his material. He showed us a pH meter with which he said he measured the pH of blood by vein. He considered the pH of blood very important. Although we all spoke German to some extent, we could not learn what type of vaccines he was using nor what his results were. In later years we were to duplicate some of the Von Brehmer methods for culturing the specific microorganisms. We also used some of his staining methods.

Dr. Von Brehmer with a group of Berlin physicians had done some outstanding work in the treatment of terminal cancer patients. He was a biologist and greatly respected throughout Europe. His vaccines for arthirtis and cancer are still in use today and are licensed by the German government. His observations, using the darkfield microscope for the examination of fresh human blood, are useful in monitoring the course of the disease. He still has many followers of his methods throughout the world today. We were to meet him in Antwerp at a later conference.

The Meetings in Rome

The Sixth International Conference of Microbiology took place in Rome from September 6–12. Scientists arrived from all over the world. Many fields of microbiology were represented. Two of the Nobel Prize winners, Sir Alexander Fleming and Dr. Selman Waksman were present. Every day in addition to the lectures there were festive events planned. We enjoyed the symphony, the art galleries, the beautiful parks and squares with their fountains, the Vatican, St. Peter's, the Tivoli Gardens. Our badges for admission to the activities were pinned with a replica of the famous wolf that nursed Romulus and Remus. We also received commemorative medals.

On September 7 in the afternoon there was a reception for all the participants at the congress and their families in the gardens of the Instituto Superiore di Sanita, the Health Department. Unlike our civic centers, the Italians surround many of their public buildings with beautiful gardens and fountains so that the people who work there can enjoy their surroundings, quite a contrast to the huge concrete parking lots surrounding our public buildings. As usual, there was lovely music, the splash of fountains, the congeniality of good food and cooling drinks. Our group was sitting at a small table when Dr. Jerome Alexander glanced up and said, "Look, children, there are three famous Nobel Prize winners standing there together. Take your cards and go over and get their autographs." Toggy and Julie went over to the three men. Two of them turned their backs on the children but Sir Alexander Fleming took each child by the hand and led them to a bench. He held Julie on his lap and put his arm around Toggy. He asked them their names and if they were enjoying themselves. Then he signed their cards. He wrote on Julie's card "To Julie with love, Alexander Fleming. 7/9/53." The English put the day before the month.

On the afternoon of September 9 our group from the Presbyterian Hospital of Newark, New Jersey, presented our papers.

In summary it can be said that these papers demonstrated the presence of the *Cryptocides* in tissues, their cultural properties, their identification as specific microorganisms, and their ability to produce pathological lesions in experimental animals. We also demonstrated that immune bodies can be produced which indicate the close relationship of these organisms to one another whether of human or animal strains, and that the so-called "viruses" of animal tumors could well be the filterable forms of these causative bacteria. In addition, these microorganisms could produce immune bodies that affect the course of the disease in the infected host.

Dr. Hiltrud Steinbart, one of the women physicians practicing in Rome, introduced herself after our lectures and invited us to her home that evening. Her specialty was the cellular type of rejuvenation that is popular and accepted in the European countries but not in the United States even today. One of the largest centers of this work is in Romania where Dr. Ana Aslan used some procaine derivatives, which were reputed to maintain small capillary circulation and so prevent aging. In addition, Aleksander A. Bogomoletz of Russia had developed an anticytotoxic serum which also was said to prevent hardening and aging of tissues. Then, of course, Dr. Steinbart described the use of human and animal embryonic cellular therapy as devised by Neihans of Switzerland. Famous people such as Somerset Maugham, the Duke of Windsor and numerous other celebrities were reputed to have received the rejuvenation regimen with great success. To me this all sounded very exciting, if not somewhat implausible. Dr. Steinbart wondered why these methods had not been adopted in the United States. I assured her that the entire practice of medicine in the United States was under rigid government control and the likelihood of introducing such programs into our country was practically zero. All we had were face-lifting operations and silicone injections into breast tissues. However, complete organ transplants at that time were unknown.

We visited Sorrento and then embarked on the *Queen Mary* from Naples. On the trip home from Naples while we were near Gibralter, the ship ran into a heavy storm. Even in such a large ship it was hard to stand up. Julie was thrown against a heavy table during the high seas and developed a severe pain over the fresh appendectomy scar. She had had an emergency appendectomy in England. She ran a high fever and could not eat. I hunted up the ship's doctor who said, "You know as much about this as I do. I can't suggest anything but since you want some penicillin, here it is." There in the midst of the tumultous sea, the injected penicillin brought down a little girl's fever and made her well. Alexander Fleming had given Julie love in more than one way.

Meantime reports of our papers had been published in several of the newspapers in the United States. We were not aware that *The New York Times,* the *Washington Post* as well as our own hometown papers would carry an account of our presentations. We were met on docking by several newspaper science writers who told us that our reports in Rome had been challenged.

New York Doctors Challenge Cancer Germ Report

A spokeman for the New York Academy of Medicine today discounted claims of a medical research team that a cancer-causing microorganism has been isolated and that it has yielded an anticancer serum in animals.

The spokesman, Dr. Iago Galdston, executive secretary of the academy's committee on medical information, said the presence of germs in cancerous tissue has been noted before, but these appear to move in after the cancer has developed.

"This is an old story and it has not stood up under investigation," he said. "Microorganisms found in malignant tumors have been found to be secondary invaders and not the primary cause of the malignancy."

The claim was made yesterday in Rome at the Sixth International Congress of Micro-biology by a New Jersey research team. They pictured cancer as a generalized disease caused by an organism in the human blood stream, and reported that rabbits and sheep inoculated with an antiserum produced "potent immune bodies." Members of the team were Dr. Virginia Wuerthele-Caspe, Dr. Eleanor Alexander-Jackson, Dr. W. L. Smith and Dr. G. A. Clark, all associated with Presbyterian Hospital in Newark.

We expected a refutation of our work, since in 1953 it was felt that cancer was not an infectious process but a metabolic or deficiency disease. The complex cycle has come around again so that almost every scientist today believes that cancer is an infection but that no specific agent has, as yet, been identified. It was not until the New York Academy of Science meetings in 1969 that we were able to present the full scope of our work to the American scientific world.

Dr. Caspe and I returned to face a crisis in Newark, New Jersey. The Patterson factory had closed due to strikes and the death of Dr. Stephen Gottfried who had worked with Dr. Caspe. At this time Dr. James Allison presented me with an alternative. Since the Black-Stevenson funds were not to be allocated for any of the work in the microbiology of cancer, he felt that he would prefer to absorb the Presbyterian Hospital Branch of Rutgers back into the University at New Brunswick. He invited me to continue with the university as associate professor with a salary, but I would be obliged to commute to New Brunswick at least twice a week. The laboratory at Presbyterian would be the source of the material from the patients but the bacteriology would be done in the future by Dr. John Anderson. In other words, Dr. Jackson would no longer be needed under the new arrangement. He said that Rutgers would continue to underwrite my applications for grants only under these conditions. I was crushed. I thought we had done an excellent job in our presentations in Rome. Dr. Allison felt that Dr. Jackson had not deferred sufficiently to Dr. Anderson in her work.

After much soul-searching I decided to continue with Dr. Jackson and to sever my connection with Rutgers. I was well aware of the difficulties involved in raising funds without university backing and particularly since the public thought we had been well-endowed by the Black-Stevenson Trust. However, I made an effort to keep the bacteriological part of the program in operation. I spoke before numerous service clubs around the state. Many private individuals came forth with gifts but it was of no use. By the time I had attended to my practice and gone about raising the money to keep the laboratory open, there was no time for further research. At the same time, on our return from Europe, the Internal Revenue department began to harass Dr. Caspe as to the source of the funds we had used on our European trip. We were told confidentially that this investigation was instigated by "Someone high up in New York in cancer." No names could be divulged. We could only guess. It is one of the abuses of our government that the Internal Revenue department leans heavily on secret informers who are paid 10 percent for any monies that are turned up in the course of an investigation. We were able to clear ourselves of these charges, but it required a large sum of money for defense and for reviewing our sources of income, which, of course, was the British government, which had paid for consultation; the money had been used for the research presentation in Europe. In the meantime, Dr. Jackson decided to go with a private firm in New York.

I was bitter, angry, and hurt by the turn of events. It seemed that on all sides I had lost. At this time Dr. Caspe was invited to develop a large cosmetic firm in Mexico City. I was anxious to go to California since my parents had retired to San Diego, where my only sister lived.

We returned to sell the house and close the office. By this time we had acquired office equipment, many books, and quite a lot of household furniture. A great many things we gave away including most of our large library. I closed the Newark Laboratory and donated to the hospital all the equipment except that earmarked by Rutgers under the grants. I took with me my personal microscope and received permission to take the hundreds of boxes of slides on the animal experiments. These were the slides which I had studied for many months. I could not bear to part with them. In fact, they are in our garage today. They are works of art, all neatly labeled and coded. I still have the code books and my painstaking readings. By now, however, the glue on the labels has come loose and the boxes are somewhat mildewed, but even yet I cannot part with them since they represent such an important part of my life.

Ten of the most productive years of my life had been spent here. I thought of the babies I had delivered, the many wounds I had sewn up, the teachers and students I had known, the clinics I had attended, the cancerous sick that I had cared for, and, above all, the laboratory for which I had held such great hopes and that was now dismantled, never to be opened again. I held tightly to Julie's hand and consoled myself with the thought that I was joining my family in California.

The trip across the country was pleasant and uneventful. It was good to be free of responsibilities. We decided to buy a house in Beverly Hills.

The Polio Experience

By the spring of 1954 I began to look for medical work. I joined the Los Angeles County Medical Society and attended meetings. I had some previous correspondence with Dr. Charles M. Carpenter, professor of infectious diseases at the University of California, Los Angeles School of Medicine. We had several pleasant meetings but his commitments did not permit him to initiate any studies in the microbiology of cancer at that time. I then looked up my father's old friend, Dr. George Griffiths of the University of Southern California. He was head of the cardiology department there and president of the American College of Physicians of which my father was a member. He has always been a particularly wonderful man, disingenuous and friendly. His is a remarkable life story. He had been born and raised in a small Amish community in Lancaster County, Pennsylvania. The Amish have been called the plain people because of their simple customs. The women wear plain dark long dresses fastened with ties in order to avoid buttons as ornamentation. Their men wear homespun clothes and wide brimmed black hats. They travel by horse and buggy because they do not believe in automobiles and new inventions such as electricity. Years later when I was to consult Dr. Griffiths about blood-vessel implants in my heart after a coronary, he consoled me by telling me that the human body can survive all kinds of problems. He showed us a deep, wide irregular scar on his right side. He said as a boy he had developed appendicitis and the appendix apparently ruptured. Since the Amish did not have much contact with the outside world, he was left in his misery. A large mass formed in his right side and he became very feverish and suffered intense pain. About this time an itinerant butcher, a pig-sticker, was making his rounds of the Amish settlement. He recognized young George's plight, sterilized his pig-sticking knife in boiling water and cut open George's side. All the pus and suppuration gushed out of his side. The wound healed by itself and he recovered. He was to grow up, to go to medical school, and become the country's leading cardiologist, traveling all over the world on international teaching assignments.

Through Dr. Griffiths I became acquainted with some of the medical staff of the University of Southern California. Little did I think at that time that my stepson, Brent Livingston, would be graduating from the USC Medical School in 1972. I met Dr. Edmund Dubos who was head of the Lupus erythematosis Clinic. Lupus erythematosis is a collagen disease closely related to scleroderma. It can involve the skin with a red, rough butterfly formation over the nose and cheeks, but much worse than the skin manifestations is the blood-vessel involvement which causes the chronic debilitating disease of the kidneys, heart and lungs. At this time Dr. Dubos was treating these cases with antimalarials and with steroids such as cortisone, which was just beginning to be known. He was very much interested in the microbiology of lupus and scleroderma and wanted me to help him in his clinics at the Los Angeles County Hospital. First, it would be necessary for me to meet Dr. Paul Starr, the dean of the medical school. Dr. Dubos set up an appointment and took me to meet Starr. Dr. Starr was most discouraging, if not rude, and said that he did not wish to become involved in the microbiology of the collagen diseases and advised Dr. Dubos to stick with the newer steroid therapies that were just being introduced. We remained friends with the Dubos family but I did not feel that I would be welcome at the clinics so I discontinued attendance.

All avenues to research medicine seemed to be closed to me, so I returned to my old profession of school doctor. I applied to the Los Angeles County School System and was immediately hired. My boss was Dr. Claire Hunsberger, an efficient, handsome woman. At first I was assigned to the general medical offices of the Board of Education, situated at the Civic Center. I was instructed in the standard procedures. Most of my work consisted of physical checkups of teachers who were requesting sick leave or who were returning to work after an illness. Also we examined the young movie stars such as Natalie Wood, at regular intervals. After I became fully acquainted with the routine, I was assigned a number of schools where I became the attendant physician. This work was interesting but I was amazed at the poor general health of the Los Angeles schoolchildren in the schools I attended—the poor teeth, the lice and scabies, the infected adenoids and tonsils, the bad posture, the lack of muscle tone and many other signs of malnutrition. I would often discuss these problems with the nurses and teachers, but aside from free lunches and supplementary milk there didn't seem to be any real solutions. Part of my assignment included a school for the mentally handicapped. The classrooms for training these handicapped children in manual skills were well-equipped and the teachers were infinitely dedicated. Although the medical work was very interesting to me and I felt useful but frustrated, I found my daily itinerary of about one hundred miles on the Los Angeles freeway systems to be exhausting. I applied for a group of schools nearer to my home. This request was granted but before the new schedule went into effect I contracted poliomyelitis. This occurred before the Salk and Sabin immunization programs were initiated. In Los Angeles polio became epidemic. There were iron lungs available for those who needed them in the infectious disease center.

One evening after working at the schools all day, I noticed that my neck was very painful. Soon I couldn't swallow and I became feverish. The pain became excruciating and I couldn't hold up my head. Also my legs and arms ached. I got a heat lamp and began to take some pain pills. Then I realized that I must have polio. I was greatly concerned for Julie's playmates who had been constantly in and out of the house. I called for a neighborhood physician who lived across the street. He came over and agreed that I had polio but he wanted a neurological consultation. The neurologist came and said that my muscles of respiration did not seem affected, nor my brain, but that I would have to report to the County Hospital for a spinal tap. I could not be hospitalized except under extreme necessity as there were not enough beds for the polio patients. I was taken into an anteroom and told to loosen and pull my clothes down to my waist and put on an openback white gown. I did this and was then placed on a stretcher and wheeled outside to join a long line of stretchers on the sidewalk and in the courtyard of the County Hospital. There were at least thirty stretchers lined up at the doors of the treatment rooms. Children, adults, doctors, lawyers, mothers, all were there for one purpose—to see if they had a positive spinal fluid which meant that the spinal cord and brain were involved in the polio infection. If the test was negative, they could go home and wait out the disease but if it was positive, they would be hospitalized for observation to be sure that they would have the use of a resuscitator and iron lung if needed suddenly. I was too sick and weak to care. After about forty minutes I was wheeled into the treatment room. A strong nurse sat me up on the edge of the stretcher with my legs dangling. I was told to bend over, then a male nurse gently pushed my shoulders forward and in just a second without pain he had inserted a needle into my spinal cord and drawn off some fluid for testing. I was wheeled outside to the other side of the building and told to wait for the verdict. In about twenty minutes the word came back that I could go home. It took me about ten days to recover from the fever and about a month before I could hold up my head without a neck brace. Our neighborhood doctor looked in on me daily. All the children who had played with Julie received protective doses of gamma globulin. I was very unpopular. Fortunately no one contracted the disease from me.

After fifty years of the practice of medicine in Pittsburgh my father had retired to San Diego. He, too, had tried various pursuits. He joined the Lions club, took classes at State College, traveled around the world, became a realtor, but he was not satisfied until he opened a small neighborhood medical office. He, too, had a remarkable boyhood. He was the son of French-German immigrants who settled in Pittsburgh before he was born in 1885. His father, William Wuerthele, became a successful businessman and my father, his older son, helped him in his business. My father dropped out of school after the sixth grade and led a life of athletic prowess winning many medals and awards for swimming, ice-skating and bicycle racing. He became the Western Pennsylvania bicycle champion. There is a gentleman living in La Jolla now, husband of one of my Pen Women sisters, who remembers my father as a young man. My father seemed like a legendary figure to the little boys who tagged after him and wanted to ride his bicycle. One of the nicest things I could hear about my father so many years ago was that he was very kind to the little boys, taught them to ride on his bicycle and bought them ice-cream cones.

One night my father and a group of his friends were sitting around talking when one of them said he would like to go to medical school. This sounded like an interesting idea to my father so he asked his friend what was needed to enroll. His friend said, "Just your high school diploma." This stopped my father for a thoughtful minute. Then one of the boys said, "Well, you know, Hermie, I have a high school diploma. I'm not planning to use it. You can have it." My father took the other boy's diploma, used ink eradicator and then artistically put his own name on the diploma. The medical school they were talking about was part of the Western University of Pennsylvania which later became the University of Pittsburgh. In those days nothing further was required to gain entrance to the medical school. He entered with a class of thirty and graduated third in his class. He was to spend the rest of his life studying and doing medical research. He became a distinguished physician and a Fellow of the American College of Physicians.

Now, at the end of his life after giving up a large clinic in Pittsburgh, he had retired to San Diego. At seventy years of age he decided to return to the practice of medicine but he didn't have a California license. This did not concern him in the slightest. He went to Sacramento and took the examinations. When he returned we asked him how he had gotten along. He said that the written part was simple but the young doctor who gave him the orals didn't know how to conduct an examination. We asked him what had happened. He said, "Young fellow, I know that you want to find out what I know about diabetes but your question won't get the full answer. Your question should be phrased differently." He then rephrased the question and gave the answer. With many recent graduates from the leading medical schools failing the California Board of Medical Examiners, he passed with ease at seventy. He then opened a neighborhood medical office in the Kensington area of San Diego. My sister gave a party in the new office for him. Mother went with him every day to help as his office girl. Dad worked about six hours daily. After awhile Mother got tired and hired another office helper for him. He was always busy and made daily neighborhood house calls. After I moved to San Diego, occasionally I would help him at the office but mostly I was busy remodeling the old house we bought, looking after Julie and Dr. Caspe when he was home, and playing a little golf and bridge with my sister while I was recuperating.

My sister, father and I had heard that there were trials of

polio vaccinations taking place outside of the United States, but soon the vaccine would be ready for our country. I knew that Dr. Samuel Goldberg of Newark had grown the polio organisms in mouse brains and that John Franklin Enders had devised some techniques for growing the virus for vaccine. Dr. William Brodie, who was a bacteriology professor of mine at Bellevue Medical School, had made a polio vaccine. After two of the children he vaccinated died, he committed suicide. Dr. Jonas Salk was selected by Basil O'Connor of the March of Dimes to prepare the polio vaccine. He was then at the University of Pittsburgh. The poliomyelitis virus was grown in a special artificial medium on the kidney tissues of a species of Rhesus monkey from India or a Cynomologus monkey from the Philippines. The virus is killed with Formalin to destroy its infectivity but the power to stimulate antibody production is not destroyed. By this method the person receiving the vaccine was immunized against poliomyelitis.

In 1955 the new polio vaccine was rushed onto the market and promptly caused among the vaccinees and their families 10 deaths and 192 cases of paralytic polio. The Cutter "incident" as the scandal was named after the company that produced most of the bad vaccine, caused the resignation of a secretary of Health, Education and Welfare, a surgeon general and a director of the National Institute of Health. As a result the NIH laboratory responsible for regulating vaccines was reorganized as the Division of Biologics Standards. Today there is a scandal raging due to charges that the potency and efficacy of commercial influenza vaccine is under question.

By a strange coincidence my sister, Dr. Lillian Ravin, my father, Dr. H. W. Wuerthele, and I were asked to administer the first Salk vaccine in San Diego County. A public grade school in the Kensington area was selected for the first pilot administration of the Salk vaccine in San Diego. The whole procedure resembled a day at the races. Nurses were busy filling syringes. Each syringe was used to give multiple doses but was flamed in between. Records were kept of the lot number on the vaccines.

Mothers with tags on their dresses were rounding up the children who were trying to sneak around the table and act as if they had a shot when they hadn't. Some of the children howled and had to be held down forcibly. In the midst of this bedlam, my father, sister and I administered the shots to the children of the school. This took up practically the entire day. We were exhausted but we felt we were pioneers in helping to conquer poliomyelitis. None of the children to whom we gave vaccines that day had a serious reaction. All of them were apparently successfully immunized. When we were prepared to leave after we had completed inoculations of several hundred children the administrator in charge asked my sister and me if we would each like a vial of vaccine to give to our own children. We accepted. On returning home that evening I gave a dose to my ten-year-old daughter, Julie. Within four hours she developed a fever of 105, her heart rate was uncountable, her respiration was rapid and faint. She became comatose. I appealed to several pediatricians by telephone. They had no suggestion to offer. I know now that pooled gamma globulin might have helped. As it was, all I could do was to put her in a cool water bath, but when she became too weak to lie in the bathtub, I kept her packed in cold towels and forced fluids into her mouth. All night I held her in my arms praying that she would live. She scarcely knew me. By morning the fever broke, leaving her weak and confused. After a few days she seemed much better, but she had difficulty in climbing stairs and when she bent over she would lose her balance. I saved the vaccine bottle and took it to San Francisco to see Dr. Ward at Cutter Laboratories who was in charge of the polio vaccine production. He confirmed the fact that the batch number of the one I had given to my daughter was the same which had infected and even killed some of the inoculated children.

It seemed that we weathered one form of disaster only to be confronted by another. Dr. Caspe had spent three-quarters of his time in Mexico for two years developing a line of cosmetics. He had been promised not only a salary but also a percentage of the business as royalties on his processes. When the entire line of cosmetics was introduced on radio and television, he was informed that he was no longer needed. All his commitments had been made in Mexico City and were not worth the paper they were written on. He fell into a state of deep depression. He seemed ill but he would not permit my father to examine him nor would he see any other doctor. I reminded him that his mother had died of diabetes and that he might be suffering from that disease. He said that he could take care of himself and wanted no medical interference. I, too, became deeply depressed and turned for help to my family. They advised me to let him work out his own problems. He made several trips back to New York but came home again after a week or two. Finally, one day he said that he wanted me to liquidate all our San Diego assets and to return to New York with him. I refused to do this since I felt that my home was now in San Diego. However, I told him that I would mortgage our home and give him all our cash assets besides borrowing a large sum of money from my father to give him the opportunity to start a consulting firm in New York. I also said that if he became established in New York we would join him there at a later time but that I would take the medical job at the San Diego Health Association in order to support Julie and return the money my father had advanced. But he was a proud man, self-confident and determined to start a new life again. He was a brilliant biochemist and held many patents in the vitamin, drug, cosmetic and dye fields. However, he was not a sociable person and preferred to be on his own most of the time. I went out to the driveway with him, kissed him good-by and stood there wiping my eyes as he drove away. I was never to see him again.

He wrote and phoned us frequently but was out of the country a large part of the time. The government of Haiti engaged him as industrial consultant and he spent a lot of time there at Port au Prince. I kept in touch with his New York friends and relatives who said that he was stimulated by his new contacts but that he was gaining weight and keeping late hours.

I began to work full time as a medical internist and diagnostician at the San Diego Health Association. After I had worked there a few months I received word that Dr. Caspe died in a hotel room while on a purchasing trip for the Haitian government in New York City. I learned later that he had complained of a boil on his neck. When his friends called to take him to dinner the next day he was found dead in his hotel room. The coroner's report showed that he died in diabetic coma brought on by an infection.

I was now nearly fifty years old. Again I had to make a fresh start in life. My health was not good. I had bouts of asthma, attacks of dizziness and a fast heart rate from the old polio attack. However, I knew that I could not become dependent on my family and that I must gather up the courage to start a new life. Dr. Chester Antos, who was medical chief at the clinic, hired me. He was chief of pediatrics and very personable and knowledgeable. I had not practiced general medicine since leaving Newark in 1953 several years before. However, there was a shortage of doctors, particularly in this prepaid type of clinic which was just getting established. The clinic was founded by Dr. Roy Stevenson, former director of the San Diego County Hospital. He felt that a clinic could be run on an insurance plan so that people in modest circumstances when confronted with catastrophic illness would not become impoverished and become state charges. This idea was highly controversial at the time and physicians practicing in this type of clinic were barred from membership in the county medical association. In a few years group-insured medicine was recognized and considered a safeguard against socialized medicine, which the American medical profession wanted to avoid, knowing what the British physicians suffered under such a system. At this time I had no other medical choice. I needed a good salary to take care of Julie and to pay off my debts. Very little of the funds Dr. Caspe had taken to New York were recoverable.

Working at the clinic was a new experience for me. It was assembly-line medicine. That is, each physician saw about fifty patients a day. We practiced good medicine but no time was lost. Everything was streamlined. An experienced nurse was assigned to me. Patients were given ten-minute appointments. Each patient was completely set up in an examining room with histories and laboratory tests completed. In the beginning it was a strain to try to assess each patient in such a short time. After a while I learned to call them back at short intervals until I had an opportunity to become better acquainted with their particular problems. With new patients, we were allowed more time. We worked on a unit system and we were supposed to keep up a certain number of units of service each month. Since I was the last doctor to be hired I was given all the least desirable night duty and holiday on-call assignments. The general doctors, of which I was one, were on call all night every third or fourth night. This meant hospital emergency-room service as well as house calls and anesthesia when needed.

Not only was I the last physician hired but I was an "older woman." I received a man's salary but I was expected to do more than the men to earn it. I knew that new physicians were hired by the group rather frequently but after a time they were dropped before tenure was established. If I was to survive in the clinic I would have to excel and not just get by. No matter what I was called upon to do, I knew I would have to do it. Often I would be late getting away for lunch. Many times I would be booked far more heavily than the men. I would glance into their offices where they were gathered smoking and discussing the baseball scores. They earned extra units by so-called consultations which were a matter of referral from one to the other without any additional work involved. When I would suggest that they might like to take some of my overflow the reply was "You don't smoke and you don't know anything about baseball. You're not one of the boys. We don't have anything in common with you." This was true so the only way I could survive was to work endlessly which I did. Soon I had the greatest number of units in the clinic for an individual physician. My patients were appreciative and grateful. The work was stimulating and I was learning new skills.

As I look back on those years I realize now that most of the diagnostic work in the clinic revolved around cancer detection. Any aberrant symptom had to be evaluated in the light of a latent cancer until it was ruled out. Cardiovascular disease, obesity, endocrine imbalances, diabetes, nervous disorders, nutritional defects, collagen diseases, gynecological problems in women, the debility of aging, family problems, all fell within the scope of my practice. But over it all fell the pall of the fear of cancer. We took Pap smears on all the women. Everyone had a complete physical on her first visit. In many ways the clinic served as a cancer detection clinic. A fever of unknown origin could turn out to be a sarcoma somewhere in the body made manifest weeks later after much laboratory work and X-rays. By then, it was already too late to do anything. Even if we had known that cancer was imminent there was no treatment. There was nothing to do but wait until a tumor presented itself and then attempt to cut it out or destroy it by radiation or chemicals. A woman might complain of pain over an ovary. Nothing could be found. After several months a small mass might develop which when operated, proved to be an ovarian cancer. Since she was carefully watched, it was detected early and was operable. I used to think, why can't we have a test that will show the neoplastic disease before the tumor develops? That possibility now exists.

Sometimes humorous situations would develop. One time a woman was coming to me to be treated for nervous symptoms. I asked her everything I could think of and checked her out completely. She seemed to be normal. As she was leaving I asked her again, "Are you sure you have told me everything?"

"Well, doctor," she said, "Could it be I am nervous because I suspect my husband is trying to kill me? I don't think he likes me."

I replied very carefully, "What makes you think that?"

"Well," she said, "there was a full bottle of Antrol in the medicine cabinet next to my almost empty cough medicine bottle. The next day the Antrol bottle was almost empty and my cough medicine was full. I was so nervous I was afraid to take it. You'd better give me another prescription."

"Anything else?" I asked.

"Yes, indeed. Look here," she held the skirt of her dress up to the light. "See, he cut the center out of every flower on the front of this dress. And it's just new, too. He cuts my shoelaces and puts sand into the Wheatena."

"It seems that you do have plenty to make you nervous. I think you'd better not go home until your daughter comes to get you. You'd better go visiting for a while until we check your husband."

On another occasion when I was on emergency night call at the clinic a man brought in his three-year-old child. I asked him what the trouble was. He said the little boy was vomiting ants. I said that was a strange complaint. Where did the little boy get the ants? I couldn't visualize his eating them from an ant hill.

"I suppose," he said crossly at my stupidity, "it must be from the bottle of Antrol he just drank."

We had a program for complete semiannual physicals for executives and professors from San Diego State College who were enrolled in the athletic fitness program. One of the procedures was a sigmoidoscope examination which involves passing an eighteen-inch telescope up the posterior of the patient after he has been suitably evacuated. Each of the doctors was scheduled to perform a certain number of sigmoidoscopic examinations each month. However, on one occasion, a problem arose. One of the professors at the State College whom I had known socially for some time was scheduled for a sigmoidoscopic with me one morning. Neither of us was aware of the other's identity. He was an extremely tall large man, head of his department. When we met he began to laugh and said he was willing if I was. We agreed that this was a very useful procedure but it would involve his standing on his head for me. He was prepared and taken into the sigmoid room and placed on the examining table, the head down with shoulders braced and the posterior pointed ceiling-ward. My nurse called me when ready. There was just one difficulty. I was too short to reach the point of operation. I couldn't even put the sigmoidoscope in place let alone look into it. We were at an impasse. Our friend was getting red in the face from standing on his head. Suddenly inspiration seized me. The maintenance man was out in the hall using a small ladder to replace a light bulb. I rushed out into the hall, brought the ladder in and triumphantly ascended it. I could assure my friend that all was well. The next time we met at a social gathering he laughed and said, "Virginia and I have a little secret but we'll never tell."

The Meetings
in Antwerp

These months at the clinic were strenuous. I could not be immobilized by grief under these circumstances. Weekends when I was free I took Julie to the zoo, to the movies, to the circus. My mother and sister lived close by and could supervise her when I was late getting back from the clinic. Often I had to leave early in the morning to administer anesthetics in the clinic. Many surgeries such as tonsillectomies and reduction of simple fractures were done there. I had not given anesthesia since my intern days but again, I could not admit to any incapability so I always approached these mornings with a certain amount of trepidation. Of course, after I had done the procedures a few times, they became routine. Until now I had not received much help or encouragement from my medical peers at the clinic. Later, when I became well-known at the clinic I was a threat to their prestige. I also developed the largest drawing and earning power in the medical department. But this was to be later. At this time the giving of several anesthetics in the early morning in addition to the usual office schedule of patients meant getting there very early. My first experience was with Dr. A. M. Livingston who was head of the eye, ear, nose, throat and allergy department. The chief nurse of the clinic, Ethel Sebetic, reassured me, "He's nice. He'll help you. Don't worry." After each child was wheeled in, sedated, I would start pouring ether by the open cone method. Some of the children struggled but gently I would try to put them to sleep. Dr. Livingston said, "Don't put them out too far, I want them to awaken as soon as I am through." He was quick and skillful. Everything always went smoothly with him. He was cheerful and competent. Gradually we got into the habit of taking our children out together on the weekends. I became very interested in the Mormon religion through him. I learned that he had been a Mormon missionary in his youth, that his family were early settlers in Utah, and that he was a priest and teacher in his church ward. I became a convert to the Mormon Church and on October 5, 1957, we were married. Now I felt that I had roots, that I had come home, that I was happy, and that I had complete confidence in this gentle, devout, kindly man. Our marriage has been a completely happy one.

It was not so difficult for me now in many ways. When it was necessary to make night calls A. M. would get up and go with me. We enjoyed our work and our home life with the children. Although I was no longer actively engaged in cancer research except in the clinical aspect of cancer detection, our papers from the Rome congress sparked a great deal of interest among other research workers all over the world. There were many other distinguished scientists who believed in the infectious nature of cancer. They had isolated the pleomorphic micro-organism which we later called *Cryptocides* and they called it by a number of different names. However, what they saw was undoubtedly some form of the same causative agent. We had no quarrel with the European investigators. I believed that I was the first investigator to show that the causative organism was an Actinomycetales, which includes the tubercle bacillus, and that the so-called "viruses" of animal tumors were, in reality, filterable forms of this same organism. Dr. Jackson's work in the pleomorphism of the lepra and tubercle bacillus greatly enhanced this concept.

Dr. Jackson, in New York, became interested in the European group and was appointed the American secretary to the First International Congress for Microbiology of Cancer and Leukemia. A congress was set up in Antwerp which is very close to Brussels. This was the year of the Brussels World Fair. The congress was held "Under the high protection of the General Commissariat of the Government at the World Exhibition." I was made one of the three vice-presidents. Dr. E. Villequez, director of the Central Blood Bank of France and professor of Experimental Medicine at the University of Dijon, France, was the president, Hofrat Professor Dr. F. Gerlach from the University of Vienna, Austria, was a vice-president also as was Doctor Clara J. Fonti, presidente del Centro Internazionale Oncological di Viggio, Milan, Italy.

My husband and I were able to arrange vacation time together from the clinic. We took the two children with us and flew to London over the Pole. We attended a cancer congress in London which was largely a discussion of therapeutics. We thought that much of the work presented there was a waste of time because the therapy was aimed at the result of the infectious process and not at the cause.

We met the Dillers at the London Congress but Dr. Jackson did not join us until we reached Antwerp. Dr. Frank van den Bosch was in charge of our arrangements in Antwerp. He met us and the Dillers at the railroad station with a fleet of small European cars apparently commandeered from among his acquaintances. We were driven to a romantic castle, now a hotel, on the shores of a woodland lake. It was a parklike place where the people of Antwerp bicycled around the lake in the evenings and weekends. Everyone bicycled. Small children who could scarcely walk got out of their perambulators and took off on tiny tricycles. Their favorite refreshment was a parfait glass of fresh fruit yogurt. These were prepared in great quantities and placed in a large iced glass showcase. I thought how much more healthful these were compared to the candy and heavily sweetened ice cream, soft drinks, and popsicles our American children are given.

The congress was a great success. Fortunately I had become quite fluent in French and German during my college years so I was able to understand most of the presentations given at the meetings. We did not have multiple translation, so we had to rely on direct communications at the various dinners and festivities.

On Monday, July 14, 1958, the congress convened. The academical opening began with an address by the president, Professor E. Villequez on "Humanism and the Struggle Against Cancer." The rest of the day was devoted to a social hour and dinner. We had the opportunity of renewing our acquaintance with doctors Gerlach and Von Brehmer. Dr. Gerlach went to Africa after leaving the United States from his visit at the Newark laboratory. Dr. Von Brehmer did not look well. He had had a leg amputed due to diabetes and looked rather thin. He has since died.

I had the honor of being the first speaker of the first day of the scientific session. The papers presented were entirely concerned with the immunologic approach to the cancer problem. Again, this material was far in advance of the work in the United States. Only recently has Dr. Robert Huebner of the National Cancer Institute's division of virology proposed the theory of the C-particle, a noncontagious virus, to be the cause of cancer when activated. This Huebner theory on which great sums of money have been expended is very old hat. At the afternoon meeting Dr. Nello Mori, Director of the Istituto Microbiologicol Bella Vista, Naples, spoke on "My Conception of the Causative-Pathological Symbiosis of a Certain Parasite in Cancer and Methods of Combating the Parasite by Immunization." Dr. Gerlach spoke on "Latency and Regression of Tumors Brought About by Specific Therapy." Dr. Clara Fonti spoke on the pathogenic etiology of cancer and its treatment. Dr. Eleanor Jackson demonstrated her film on the "Morphological Changes in the Human Tubercle Bacillus." Dr. Diller spoke on the "Morphological Changes in Mouse and Rat Blood."

All of these distinguished scientists had been carrying on research in the biological and immunological treatment of cancer for years. It is only now that the United States is beginning to catch up. Because of the suppressive action of the American Cancer Society, the American Medical Association and the Federal Drug Administration, our people have not had the advantage of the European research. Also, the deliberate suppression of our work in this country has set cancer research back a number of decades.

However, if the animal immunization studies done by Shope, Andervont, Bittner and others in this country had been regarded as prototypes for human immunization, and the early work of Glover, Gregory, and L'Esperance had been taken more seriously, cancer treatment would now be far advanced. This work has been ignored because certain powerful men backed by large monetary grants can become the dictators of research and suppress all work that does not promote their interests and that may present a threat to their prestige.

Of particular interest to me was the work of Dr. Clara J. Fonti of Milan. In the autumn 1958 her book called, *Eziopatogenesi del Cancro* was published by Amedeo Nicola & C. Milano. It was dedicated "Alla memoria del Dott. Amelio Fonti, Compagno della mia vita, apostolo dei malatti e dei poveri—con amore." "To the memory of Dr. Amelio Fonti, companion of my life, apostle of the sick and of the poor—with love." In the foreword she further writes, "Agli studiosi di tutto il mondo perche continuino il mio lavoro e lo perfecionino per amore della scienza e dell' umanita." "May the students of the world continue with my work to perfection through love of science and of humanity." This remarkable woman not only developed a method of staining preserved blood slides so that the presence of the cancer infection could be evaluated in the blood of patients but she generously gave all of her knowledge of her procedures and treatment in this book. It is painstakingly written with great accuracy and has many beautiful colored illustrations. What impressed me above all is her Chapter III on *Autocontagio*, or Self-infection. She was a ponderous, stout, stately Italian woman. In 1959 Dr. Fonti inoculated the skin on her chest between her breasts with a cancer culture—not with the cells but with the culture. A cancerous growth occurred in the area. This Dr. Fonti removed and had analyzed. The diagnosis revealed that a cancer had been produced through the inoculation of a *bacterial culture*. There is a photograph of the lesion as well as a photomicrograph of the pathological section with the diagnosis of a "basal cell epithelioma." All of us who have studied the microbiology of cancer are convinced that the disease is infectious and not contagious, that is, that it can be transmitted by direct contact.

The Brussels Fair was a great experience for us. Since we were honored guests we did not have to wait at any of the exhibits but could get into the pavilions immediately. Dr. Frank van den Bosch who was our principal host was exhibiting a computing ultraviolet microscope at the Bell Laboratories Pavilion. It had a magnification of 30,000 and did not destroy the material which was under examination. The electron microscope kills the specimens and photographs them in an inert state whereas this microscope preserved them in their living condition and they could be projected on to a television screen where they could be photographed. It also had a computer attachment which permitted the counting of blood cells and microorganisms. Dr. van den Bosch also developed an electronic device which, on being attached to the visual centers of the brain, acted as receptors or eyes for the blind. Later, my husband and I were to finance a trip for him to the United States where he lectured on his optical receptor at the San Diego Biomedical Society. His work was greeted with skepticism here but ten years later, similar work was initiated in the United States. He is now at the Downstate Medical

Center of the University of the State of New York in Brooklyn.

During this time my father became very ill and vomited blood. He had X-rays taken and was told that he probably had cancer of the stomach. He was admitted to Mercy Hospital where he was scheduled for surgery the following day. Since I had become a member of the Mormon Church I had seen a number of examples of people being cured of their illness by the power of prayer. I was so distressed for my father that I asked my husband and Patriarch Clinger of the Church to come to the hospital to administer to him. This is done by anointing the head of the sick person with oil that has been sanctified; a prayer is then offered by those who are authorized to do so to heal the sick according to the will of the Lord in the name of Jesus Christ. I thought that this was my father's last day on earth and I was crying bitterly. My husband offered the opening prayer and then Brother Clinger blessed him. He turned to me and said, "Dry your eyes, Sister Livingston, your father is well. Nothing will be found wrong with him tomorrow at surgery."

I looked at Patriarch Clinger's calm, spiritual face in astonishment. "How do you know?"

He patted my shoulder and said, "I know."

The next morning about eleven o'clock when my mother, sister Lillian, and I were in the lunchroom getting my mother some tea, my name was called on the loudspeaker to come to the operating room at once. I jumped up nervously and ran out of the room. When I arrived at the surgery, I was asked to wait for Dr. Brown.

Dr. Maurice Brown, chief of the Mercy staff of surgeons, said to me, "We have opened your father from the pelvis all the way up to his chest. We have opened his stomach also. There is absolutely nothing the matter with him. Yet only yesterday a large mass was present in his stomach both by examination and by X-rays. Would you like me to take out his stomach anyway?"

"No, no," I said, "not if everything looks all right."

Dr. Brown said, "I still can't understand it but we'll just close him up."

"Please do that," I said. "My father had a blessing last night and I was told that he was healed." Dr. Brown walked away without any further comment. My father lived eight more years, without recurrence of the stomach problem.

The work at the clinic became more demanding all the time. The other physicians resented my husband and me because we were drawing down a double maximum salary. True, my husband's department was the most lucrative and I had the largest patient load in the medical department, yet the jealousy was there. Sometimes when I had been up all night with a particularly sick patient I would have difficulty in getting one of the men to take over promptly in the morning so that I could get some sleep. In February of 1962 I had put in an extremely difficult week. An elderly lady, a member of our church, had been very ill and I had spent extra time with her. I was very tired but still carrying on daily. It would probably have been better if we have left the clinic but we were helping Rodney Livingston through dental school at Baylor University. He had married a nonworking wife so we had a heavy load with his tuition and dental supplies. We felt it would be better to stick it out until he was through school. At any rate, on this particular early afternoon my heart appeared to stop. I had no pulse and became extremely weak. I had my nurse call my husband from his office. He came upstairs promptly. I told him that I was having a serious heart attack but that I wanted to leave the clinic and go to a cardiologist that I knew in La Jolla. We told my nurse to notify the others that we were leaving. Then we went down the back stairs to our car and my husband drove me to Dr. David Carmichael's office in La Jolla. Dr. Carmichael took us in immediately. The cardiogram showed that I had almost no heart beats at all. He gave me some medication and then sent my husband to the pharmacy in the same building. Dr. Carmichael sat in the car with me. I saw two tears roll down his cheeks. It surprised me when he said, "You know you could be dying. You don't have any pulse or any beats."

I replied, "I don't think so. I'll be all right. I just need rest."

My husband took me to the hospital where I spent ten of the most miserable days of my life. There was no private room and I was given a bed in a room with a woman who was throwing a good-by party for her friends and nurses with cake and ice cream, because she was being discharged that afternoon. No one paid the slightest attention to me. Finally, a nurse answered the buzzer and I asked her to remove the party as I was very ill.

She said, "When you get this hypo, you won't care."

I said, "What hypo?"

"You're not supposed to know, but since you are a doctor it's morphine ordered for every three hours."

I said, "No morphine for me. Get those people out of here and let me sleep."

I slept with a mild sedative. The next day I was moved to a private room with private nurses. I became extremely short of breath and had a blue cyanotic color. I could breathe only under oxygen. When things became unbearable, the Elders from the church came and administered to me. Now at least I could breathe. The food was atrocious. All canned fruit, white potato mix, coffee, white cheap bread, hamburger, jello. Ever since this experience I have urged my patients who are hospital bound to be sure that their friends and relatives are permitted to bring them "hospital care packages" to consist of fresh fruit and vegetable juices. Also a supply of good bread, fresh butter, cheese and their usual vitamins. Many hospitals feed the patients on "convenience food," that is food that is prepared in bulk or frozen and packaged ahead and that is heated up by electronic ovens or infrared heating units just before serving. The hospital dietitians are more concerned with the fat, carbo-hydrate, protein and total calorie count that with the quality of the food. A long stay in a typical hospital could lead to devitaminosis and a loss of essential enzymes, minerals and food factors not present in processed and preserved foods. I was grateful that during my hospital stay one of my friends brought me several care packages containing the essential vitamins and a good supply of vitamin E. I was discharged in ten days, but now I was a cardiac cripple.

A nurse was in constant attendance for one month. A tank of oxygen was beside my bed. I couldn't clothe or feed myself without turning purple. The slightest exertion caused me to pant. After a month, we engaged a full-time nurse-companion for me who was to stay with us for two years. Her name was Bernice Kraus and she was a member of the Church. She came every morning before my husband left and stayed until he returned. I could not walk at all and had to be pushed around in a wheel chair. Fortunately the year before the heart attack we had moved to a ranch-style house. Now I began to knit, crochet, and watch television. The days seemed endless. Finally, I decided that I was not going to sit on a couch for the rest of my life. I applied for the job of teaching a course in Mental Health and Hygiene at Calwestern University. I did not mention my disability but just said I was retired from medical practice. Two days a week I lectured to the classes. Bernice hauled me over in the car and helped me into the classroom. I could not stand up from the desk to write on the blackboard so Bernice prepared the material on the board. Fortunately it was a noncontroversial course and not difficult to teach so that it relieved the boredom of my days. Meantime I was taking enormous doses of vitamin E and other vitamins as well as adhering to a strict diet of fresh foods low in fats and sugars. We consulted the leading cardiologists in San Diego and Los Angeles. We saw Dr. George Griffiths who recommended an internal mammary artery transplant. After I read the survival statistics I was not greatly impressed. Since then there has been considerable improvement in coronary artery implants now using the saphenous vein from the leg. However, at the time, I decided to try to survive by other methods.

During this period, when I began to be a little better, I reread many of the papers we had written in the past. I was impressed by the fact that many of our experimental animals that survived cancer developed interstitial collagen disease as a result of their inoculations with our bacterial isolates of *Cryptocides* and also developed heart lesions. Even baby mice born of infected mothers often died and the autopsy showed destruction of heart muscle. These lesions contained the acid-fast organisms in the heart muscle. Eleanor wrote to me and offered to make me a vaccine in accordance with the method of Dr. Crofton in England. She thought it might do me some good. Also, a number of research people in England were reporting strange microbic bodies in the hearts of people who died of coronary disease. I had a cancer of the forehead treated successfully with radium fifteen years previously so I knew that I was a latent carrier of the *Cryptocides*. Eleanor made me a vaccine according to the Crofton method and I have had a new one every year and have continued vaccine intermittently until the present time.

We wrote a paper together called "Mycobacterial Forms in Myocardial Vascular Disease" which was published in 1965. It proposes the theory that there are microbic bodies in the lesions of heart diseases and that they are especially numerous in the areas where the blood vessels have ruptured. Until recently the theory has been that coronary blood vessels of the heart are narrowed due to arteriosclerosis, and that fatty deposits in the walls of the vessels and overweight are the determining factors in this type of heart disease. Now the medical researchers are becoming aware of the fact that the blood vessels themselves are often not involved so much as the supporting tissues and muscles of the heart so that the heart vessels rupture due to extrinsic factors outside the vessel rather than from intrinsic disease. This is particularly true of patients with collagen diseases such as scleroderma and lupus erythematosis. A reprint of the paper follows:

Mycobacterial Forms in
Myocardial Vascular Disease

Virginia Wuerthele-Caspe Livingston, M.D.,
and Eleanor Alexander-Jackson, Ph.D.

During the intervening decade from 1954-1964, we have continued our individual research and observation of certain plemorphic intermittently acid-fast micro-organisms in various proliferative, degenerative, and neoplastic diseases of man and animals. During the past year, we have re-united our efforts in a study of vascular and myocardial pathology as possibly related to chronic low-grade infection by these mycobacterium-like organisms.

In the early years of our collaboration, the work was largely focused on the identification of submicroscopic virus size bodies (20-70mμ), visualized in the electron microscope, and their relationship to larger mycobacterial forms consistently observed in and cultured from neoplastic disease. The original papers explored the occurrence of these bodies in tissues, their cultural properties and means of identification, and the pathologic conditions produced experimentally in laboratory animals. Protection studies by production of rabbit immune serum in which antitumor sera and antibacterial isolate sera against fowl leukosis were compared were attempted on a small but successful scale.

During the years when production of neoplastic lesions was predominately pursued, accompanying widespread degenerative lesions were noted. Why neoplastic disease should predominate in some animals while degenerative lesions are more prominent in others is not understood. It is the purpose of this paper to demonstrate degenerative changes occurring in coronary heart disease in the presence of invasive mycobacterial parasites. These organisms, which appear primarily as small acid-fast granules in young cultures, and which tend to become non-acid-fast in the larger forms present in older cultures, may exhibit a number of morphologic phases with intermediate transitional forms. These include (1) filterable and submicroscopic bodies; (2) larger granules readily visible under the light microscope and often resembling ordinary micrococci; (3) larger globoidal cystlike bodies and thin-walled sacs containing the smaller forms; (4) PPLO or L type zoogleal symplasms without cell walls; (5) rods of various sizes capable of developing a characteristic motility; (6) long filaments and threads which may show lateral branching; and (7) thick-walled spore-like bodies. The lesions produced by these organisms in experimental animals were generally pseudocaseous, degenerative in type, occasionally neoplastic, and occurred principally in the liver, kidneys, and lungs although, at times, there was involvement of the heart, spleen, adrenal glands, stomach, lymph nodes, and omentum.

With the preceding studies as a basis for further investigation, postmortem heart sections of 6 patients with coronary and aortic disease were stained by the Fite modification of the Ziehl-Neelsen technique (for demonstrating Lepra bacilli in sections) using Kinyoun's carbol-fuchsin, and compared with sections of the same involved areas stained with conventional H and E. Eight predominant types of lesions were observed in the myocardium.

1. PERIVASCULAR CHANGES AROUND THE SMALL CORONARY VESSELS. In the loose connective tissues numerous small acid-fast bodies can be seen.

2. CELLULAR INFILTRATION. This is frequently seen not only around the vessels but between the muscle fibers as well. These cells consist almost entirely of mononuclear types, predominantly lymphocytes, while large mononuclear phagocytes laden with organisms in both granular and coccobacillary forms are prominent; plasma and other mononuclear cells are present in relatively large numbers.

3. FIBROBLASTIC INFILTRATION. The presence of these organisms appears to stimulate the formation of fibroblasts. In some areas, the muscle fibers and interstitial tissues appear to be replaced by fibroblasts.

4. INFARCTION. Where there has been an infarct, there may be a softened central area with numerous small acid-fast cocci and coccobacilli present in the collagenous hemorrhagic softened area.

5. NECROSIS. Necrotic changes may involve the blood vessels. Striking degenerative changes of the vessel walls are observed as illustrated not only by the sections of coronary vessels but also by the sections of an involved aorta. Proliferative changes may involve the endothelium, with invasion of the endothelial cells, and are accompanied by thickening and narrowing of the wall. Hairlike filaments of the organisms were seen protruding into the lumen. These changes are also present in the vasa vasorum of the aorta.

6. THROMBOSIS AND RECANALIZATION. Some areas of recanalization were observed in heart, liver, and spleen.

7. CHANGES IN THE ELASTIC LAYER OF THE AORTA. The elastic fibrils have lost their identity and have become collagenized with loss of structure. As scar tissue forms, cholesterol-like plaques occur. It seems possible that deposits may be derived in part from the fatty envelopes of these organisms. In other tissues where masses of the organisms have proliferated, polyhedral crystals resembling cholesterol have been observed.

8. CHANGES IN THE HEART MUSCLE. Individual nuclei of the heart muscle are frequently parasitized, and replaced by small acid-fast globoidal bodies. The muscle fibers themselves appear in a state of gradual digestion and disintegration by both minute and larger acid-fast forms.

The papers of Papez describe the presence of similar bodies, which he observed unstained, in material from cerebrovascular disease associated with various types of psychoses. He states: "Sclerotic patches were found to consist of numerous mycotic cells surrounded by thick walls of cholesterol. This gave the patches the appearance of aggregates of lipofuscin granules." The pathological changes described by him appear to resemble the vascular involvement observed in our studies of myocardial disease. . . .

The American Cancer Society Meetings

During the years that I was recovering from a serious heart ailment, Dr. E. A. Jackson received a grant from the National Institute of Health (NIH) to continue with the Rous work at the Institute of Comparative Medicine at the College of Physicians and Surgeons of Columbia University. In the meantime, Dr. Irene Diller and her colleagues at the Institute for Cancer Research in Philadelphia were carrying on corroborative studies of the acid-fast organisms I had first described in 1947. As stated previously, although these specific microorganisms later called P. *Cryptocides* were observed for more than two hundred years in one or another of their various forms, it was not until I demonstrated that they are acid-fast and related to the tuberculosis family of microbes that they became readily demonstrable in tissues and cultures. Prior to 1951 Dr. Diller had been working with fungi in tumor tissue. In 1951 she began to perform isolation studies mainly concerned with an attempt to reconcile her findings with those reported by myself, Glover,

Gerlach and Villequez. From this time forward Dr. Irene Diller studied these acid-fast organisms which I initially called *Mycobacterium tumefaciens humanis,* the human strain. Later, we were asked to modify this classification and reclassify them into a separate group since in some ways the strains differ from other mycobacteria. This classification was presented in 1969 as Progenitor *Cryptocides* under the Actinomycetales, species *Cryptocides tumefaciens* including rat, bird, mouse and human strains. Dr. Diller's papers were corroborative in every respect. She studied the occurence of the *Cryptocides* in animals and received human strains for comparison. She induced disease in the mice and also was able to demonstrate the presence of the organisms in the blood of the tumor-bearing mice in a predictive way, that is, she could predict which mice would develop cancer. One of her classical papers is appended to the end of this book.

In 1965 Dr. Irene Diller was invited to attend the annual American Cancer Seminar for Science Writers that was held in New Orleans that year. True to character, Irene gave a fair and impartial presentation of the microbiological approaches to the cancer problem in which we had all collaborated. On March 30, 1965, I was made aware of her report by an article which appeared in the *San Diego Union.* As a result of Irene's presentation, Eleanor and I were invited to present papers at the 1966 seminar that was held March 25-30 at Del Webb's Town House in Phoenix, Arizona. These seminars were initiated as a means of advising the tax-paying, gift-donating public as to what is being done with the money invested in cancer research. "Between the exhilaration of the fine work presented and the relaxed atmosphere of the meeting which is planned with ample time for social pleasures, the seminars are enjoyable as well as educational." The inviting letter was signed by Dr. Harold S. Diehl, Senior Vice President for Research and Medical Affairs. He has always been a gentle, kindly man. We also knew that our old-time friend, Patrick McGrady would be in charge of the science writers and their scheduled releases. My husband,

Dr. A. M. Livingston, was generously invited to attend with us. It is considered a great honor to be invited to become a member of the "faculty" of the seminar. Thereafter the names of the participants are kept permanently on the Faculty Roster.

It was, indeed, a stimulating and interesting occasion. In fact, it was a most unique experience. Here we were at a fine hotel having a wonderful time as guests of the American Cancer Society with no obligation on our part except to participate in the Science Seminar. We were taken to a reception at Senator Barry Goldwater's house and to the country club. Every day after the science sessions there was a social hour. Since we are nondrinkers it was a source of amazement to us to see the amount of liquor consumed. Between sessions in the daytime it was very pleasant to sit around the pool and to make the acquaintance of other participants. Mr. McGrady told A. M., Eleanor and me that we would be on the program for the last day since our material was quite controversial and he thought there would be less commotion after our presentation at that time.

This timing of our presentation was undoubtedly wise. Whenever anyone presents a new concept and criticizes the old ones then the proposer must be prepared to stand the "slings and arrows of outrageous fortune." I knew what would happen when we stood on the podium and offered our papers. Eleanor was in a relatively safe position because she was discussing the immunization of chickens against Rous sarcoma with the use of bacterial isolates derived from the Bryan strain of the Rous tumor agent, erroneously called a virus. Her work was a continuation of our Rutgers studies and she had followed up with an intensive, well-controlled job of fowl immunization. I, on the other hand, was placed in the position of proposing new methods of immunologic treatment of cancer in humans. I felt like the bull's eye in the target of a dart game. Before going to the podium I took the opportunity of slipping away to the ladies' room where I fortified myself with a mild sedative and a heart pill. Then I offered up a silent prayer that there would be ears to hear and minds and hearts that would open to our message.

I had intended only to present the theoretical aspects for determining the cancer-prone individual and to suggest future methods for preventive immunization. Also, I wanted to convince our scientific audience that cancer is an infection and that surgery, radiation and chemicals cannot eradicate a continuing infectious process. I stated that "a screening program of the entire population could be undertaken by routine blood cultures to determine the presence of these mycobacteria, correlated with evaluation of blood smears and related to immune competency by various methods of antigen-antibody determination." Both of us claimed that this organism had the ability to change its form and might vary its appearance from that of a fungus to that of a cluster of virus-size pluero-pneumonialike organisms, PPLO, or Mycoplasma. I had not intended at that time to discuss some of my earliest efforts in immunizing patients. When I was asked if that were possible I replied that it was and cited three early cases. Immediately the press misquoted us and said we had a cure for cancer by immunization when that was not our main objective in the presentation of our work. I stated that the collagenophilic mycobacteria, which include the cancer organism, have thrown researchers off for years because they are able to change their forms. I also reported that in a series of breast-cancer studies at the Naval Hospital in San Diego, the best results were obtained with surgery alone, the next best with surgery and radiation, and the worst with surgery, radiation and chemicals. I implied that the cobalt machine might reduce the size of the tumors but contributed very little to the long-term cure of the disease. Dr. John Lawrence of the Lawrence Radiation Laboratories had previously stated that his hope was for a cobalt machine in every town and village in the United States. At that statement, I became excited and began to wave a Petri dish (used for making cultures) over my head and said that it could be mightier that all the high-powered radiation machines in the world. Nice Dr. Diehl tried to smooth over this statement by saying that

"Thousands of patients have been cured by surgery and radiation but of course we hope that research will eventually render these treatments unnecessary."

The Phoenix newspapers were kind, also, and reported our "basic requirements for formation of the cancer cell to be the causative microorganism and that all other factors such as coal-tar irritants, other microorganisms, the aging process, any chronic irritants leading to poor local resistance and giving rise to immature, susceptible reparative cells, may prepare the soil for the multiplication of the cancer organism and its penetration into the cyptoplasm and nucleus of the host cell." One of the officials of the cancer society (Patrick K. McGrady) said, "It could be they are right. Cynicism has never cured cancer and never will." Dr. Jorgen Fogh, a virologist at the Sloan-Kettering Institute for Cancer Research in New York said in an interview that he had examined more than 150 cancers including a dozen leukemias and had found nothing that resembled mycoplasma or the PPLO. Meanwhile, Dr. Leon Dmoschowski of the University of Texas, M.D. Anderson Hospital and Tumor Institute, was coming up with evidence that mycoplasma may, indeed, play a part in cancer. The emphasis as to which point of view is favored depends on the prestige of the institution rather than on the merits of the research.

Three years later in the *Journal of the American Medical Association,* July 28, 1969, Vol. 209, No. 4, there was a summary of the work of K. A. Bisset who wrote in the *New Scientist,* June 12, 1969, that, "Various Mycoplasma have been suspected of causing some disease whose etiology is not yet clear." He speculates that many diseases like leukemia and arthritis could be caused by Mycoplasma or by parts of this elusive bacteria. "The fact that Mycoplasma can break down into viruslike particles, easily identifiable on electron-microscope examination and similar to those found in blood of leukemia patients, leads to a strong suspicion that Mycoplasma may be a culprit in the development of certain malignant processes." Also a recent statement by Dr. Bernard Roswit reporting at Chicago the year-long study of more than five hundred patients at seventeen Veterans' Administration hospitals at the Radiological Society of North America states that "At present it appears that the patient is at the mercy of his cancer and his survival depends more upon the stage of the disease, type of cell and biological character of the cancer than upon the therapeutic act." The patients were divided into two groups, half receiving the best of radiation treatment and the other half only sugar pills. At the end of the year only 18 percent of the radiated were alive while 14 percent of those getting sugar pills alone survived. Those treated lived only thirty days longer than the untreated and none of the patients in either group was cured. However, he said the radiation did shrink the tumors temporarily and helped the morale of the patients but it did not prolong life.

There was a sad aftermath to the Cancer Seminar Meeting for Eleanor. Someone of the Cancer Society or affiliates who was high up in the hierarchy called the dean at Columbia University and had Eleanor's work terminated there. All people who inquired concerning my work were told that my results were "unproven." By whom? No one ever came to ask for case records or to interview patients. This kind of thing could appear to be a part of the great conspiracy to keep cancer research funds in the hands of a favored few who wield repressive, dictatorial, and destructive power over anyone who does not goose-step to the tune played by the dictators of American cancer politics. There are some good men in these organizations, of course, but they are not part of the power group that seeks to dictate what kind of treatment every physician shall prescribe and what every patient must receive. A general uniformity is being forced upon the American public. If the doctor does not conform, he can lose his hospital privileges. If the patient does not conform, his insurance carriers may refuse to pay his insurance. Is not each individual a thinking being? Does he not have the right to decide what he or anyone else may do to his body? In some hospitals patients have been put on double "blind studies" where neither they nor their physicians know what they are getting. In certain cases, the cancer victims have been forced to wear wigs so that no one will know whether a drug is causing their baldness. They are herded like sheep into pens for medical treatment about which they are neither informed nor consulted.

Have we not abrogated one of our Constitutional rights?

The Constitution of the Republic should make special provision for Medical Freedom as well as Religious Freedom. To restrict the art of healing to one class of men and deny equal privileges to others will constitute the Bastille of medical science. All such laws are un-American and despotic. They are fragments of monarchy and have no place in a republic.

Benjamin Rush, M.D.
Surgeon General of the Continental Army of the United
    States
Signer of the Declaration of Independence

Cancer
in the Chicken
and the Egg:
Leukosis
in Every Pot

Television viewers in the spring of 1972 in Southern California have watched the burning of thousands upon thousands of chickens because of the epidemic of Newcastle disease in poultry. Successful vaccination has been accomplished for this disease in the past, but recently a new strain has swept California leading to the death of great numbers of birds. The new strain may be compared to the outbreak of new types of influenza among humans. Newcastle disease is said not to affect humans except in the case of poultry handlers or people with cuts in their hands. The symptoms in man are comparable to mild flu and may cause conjunctivitis or redness of the eyes. These are not particularly serious symptoms but most thinking people are reluctant to eat anything that is diseased if only mildly or remotely dangerous to man. The price of eggs and chickens has dropped in the past few weeks. On visiting the meat market, and certain self-service restaurants where food is on display for selection, large stacks of chickens are left because of the public reluctance to eat the infected fowl even though cooked and said to be harmless for man.

However, Newcastle disease, although killing thousands of chickens, is not nearly the threat to human life and disease as are the cancerous diseases in poultry. The *Wall Street Journal* of February 10, 1970, said that "Chicken Cancer Called Widespread Enough to Pose 'Nightmares' for Poultry Industry." A controversy erupted in January 1971 over how safe it is to eat diseased chickens. At that time an Agriculture department advisory panel's report had suggested relaxing federal inspection standards for poultry affected by leukosis-complex (cancer) diseases. It was contended that there isn't any known connection between the leukosis viruses and human health.

As we have demonstrated in preceding chapters, the "virus" of cancer whether of man, bird, or animal really isn't a virus in the strict sense of the word. Peyton Rous, the father of the theory of infectivity of chicken cancer, did not claim the Rous infectious material to be a virus. He always emphasized that it was a "tumor agent," because it did not need living cells to survive but could be dried and stored at room temperature and reactivated months or years later by being placed into solution and injected into susceptible chickens. In the early days of our original research at the Presbyterian Hospital under Rutgers University I felt that the Rous tumor is a prototype for all other tumors of men and animals. This is the reason we spent several years growing out the tumor agent in synthetic culture media. A virus will not grow except in the presence of living cells. We were able to grow the Rous tumor agent in sterilized beef broth that contained suitable nutrients for bacterial growth. We traced its growth pattern through all of the bacteriological stages. We knew that the infectious agent passed through filters that permitted only the passage of so-called viruses. We filtered the cultures, not the extracts of the tumors, through bacteria-restraining filters and studied these with the electron microscope with Dr. Hillier at Princeton as previously described. Then we kept the cultures in which there did not appear to be any visible form of life, incubated them at 37ºC, and from these seemingly clear broths with the agent in them, there arose the bacterial and fungal stages of the *Cryptocides*. We performed this experiment not once but dozens of times until Dr. Hillier was satisfied that we had ruled out contamination that might account for the bacterial growth on incubation. It was a tedious but exciting process to learn that a so-called virus could and did convert to a bacterium that had not only submicroscopic forms but also bacillary, coccal or round forms, and that could also develop funguslike stages and spores. On studying the growth of the tubercle bacillus, these stages were entirely comparable with the *Cryptocides*.

When we examined the cultures obtained from human cancers, there was no discernible difference in the growth pattern. The growth pattern of the chicken cancer isolates and that of man were the same. They grew in the same kind of broth in the same way and they appeared the same in chicken and human tissues. They had the same staining properties with the Ziehl-Neelsen dye. We then did the sheep immunization studies in which we found significant cross-agglutination between the Rous sarcoma, fowl leukosis and various strains of human cancers. When we injected the isolated cultures into mice, the same kind of diseased lesions developed as demonstrated in the papers in the Appendix. The Rous isolates had to be readapted to chicken tissues by passage on the allantoic membrane of fertile eggs and then replanted into young chicks. We also carried on immunization of rabbits with the leukosis agent and used the antiserum to cure chickens dying of fowl leukosis. In every way the Rous agent appeared to be a prototype for human cancer.

The Rous studies led to the cultivation of the same kind of microorganisms from other animal tumors. These invariably grew and appeared similar to the Rous and human strains. Sometimes there were differences in size or different sugar or oxygen requirements for cultivation, but essentially they were the same basic structures. These filtrates, tumor agents, or "viruses" on electron microscopy appeared basically the same. They appeared identical with the mouse-leukemia virus particles in a leukemic male mouse injected with Ludwik Gross virus-induced leukemia. They are identical to all appearances with the isolates obtained by us. Our isolates range in size from 30-100 micromu. The Gross particles are 100 micromu in the illustration. The C-particles described by Robert Huebner appear to consist of the basic form of the organism, the round or coccus stage which is always seen on all cultures and may be seen budding from the surface of infected cells. These particles are seen in great abundance in the bloods of the infected human host as shown by direct darkfield microscope examination of fresh untreated blood.

Viruses have been classified as containing either deoxyribonucleic acid DNA or ribonucleic acid RNA. The basic composition, however, of all of these particles is the same as revealed in the 1930s by Wendell Stanley, Nobel laureate of the University of California. In other words, the basic life stuff is the same whether bacterium, virus, man or mouse. Since this composition is also virtually the same as that of the gene, it is not surprising that scientists have come to regard viruses as central to the study of genetics, indeed as the key to the secret of life. The reader is referred to the book by James D. Watson, *The Double Helix,* describing how the discovery by Watson and Francis Crick led to the knowledge of the structure of DNA, a major scientific advance, which won them a Nobel Prize. Some of the chicken "viruses" are classified as DNA and some as RNA. The Rous sarcoma virus has been classified as an RNA virus. However, if the Rous agent is not a virus, then there should be both RNA and DNA in the tumor agent as there are in bacterial growths.

E. A. Jackson's paper on the "Ultraviolet Spectrogramic Microscope Studies of Rous Sarcoma Virus Cultured in Cell Free Medium" demonstrates that there is DNA present in the Rous tumor agent. Since DNA is the master molecule of heredity it has been easy for virologists to speculate on how a

DNA virus could transform normal cells to cancerous, but they could not understand how an RNA virus could do this. It seems now that RNA can direct the formation of DNA and probably vice versa. This was also proven by H. M. Temin. An enzyme has been found that transcribes the RNA virus message into DNA. It is called polymerase transcriptase.

In summary, it can be said that RNA carries the DNA message into the cytoplasm around the nucleus of the cell and directs the manufacture of enzymes and other proteins that are necessary for cell function. During cell division the DNA molecules replicate themselves exactly and the duplicate set enters the chromosomes, the storehouse for material to produce new daughter generations. Any damage to RNA base could alter the chemical activities of the cell, if the defect was transmitted to the DNA. Such a defect could cause a permanent alteration in future generations of cells. Radiation and chemicals possibly induce cancer that way and so may tumor agents. DNA's genetic message is spelled out by four chemical subunits called bases, that can be arranged in an almost infinite variety of sequences along the molecule. Each DNA molecule in a cell nucleus acts as a template or pattern for the formation of a closely similar molecule of RNA which then becomes the messenger into the cytoplasm of the cell. This DNA polymerase, as the enzyme is called, has been found to be present in large amounts in animal tumors and in man with leukemia. It may provide a test for the rapid synthesis of protein. However, the discovery of the enzyme and its blockage probably will not provide a quick cure or even any cure at all for cancer since the same enzymes are present in normal young cells grown in tissue. In other words, the enzyme may be necessary for the rapid reproduction of living cells no matter what the cause of their rapid growth, perhaps even for normal repair after an injury.

All of this knowledge of the helical structure of proteins sheds some light on the formation of cells. However, those scientists who do not believe cancer to be a wildly growing, autonomous cell do not put as much reliance upon upsetting or preventing the multiplication of the cancer cell for the cure of the disease as they do upon finding the agent that triggers off the infection that results in the cancer cell. If that agent can be destroyed and the body of the host has a high enough level of immunity both of the blood serum and of fixed and circulating tissue cells, then the cancer cell may be destroyed no matter what the genetic pattern may be. The genetic pattern may be more deranged than permanently altered. At any rate the chicken agents such as those causing myeloblastosis, considered to be RNA viruses, are shipped all over the world from the laboratory of Dr. and Mrs. Joseph Beard at Duke University for the studies of protein synthesis mediated by the enzyme transcriptase. These tumor agents have an enormous amount of activity in the synthesis of tumor agents from the cells of the young chicken. The DNA acts as a printing press which prints out RNA instructions and sends them as a messenger from the nucleus to the cell constituents giving them orders as to how to conduct their affairs.

The chicken normally has a body temperature of 105 degrees. Many of the ordinary pathogens to which man is susceptible are not a problem in the chicken. However, the mycoses, viruses and fungal diseases are prevalent in fowl. Avian lymphomatosis, or avian cancer, is a disease characterized by the accumulation of undifferentiated lymphocytes in the nerves, viscera or iris. This disease is known as neurolymphomatosis, leukemia, fowl paralysis, big liver. It is now called Marek's disease after the Hungarian pathologist who first described it in 1907. It is prevalent in many parts of the world. Of the 176,000,000 fryers slaughtered in November 1969, 2,000,000 were condemned for leukosis by inspectors. This represents an enormous loss of revenue for the poultry industry. Specialists say virtually all chickens harbor these so-called viruses and when the chicken's tissues fight back, tumors develop. The poultry industry has been asking for a relaxation of the government controls. The advisory panel recommended that the tumors be cut off the birds and the unaffected parts sold. The tumorous material could then be ground up for hot dogs for children. Dr. Bruce W. Calnek of Cornell University who is a veterinary researcher says, "We have no evidence of danger to humans and think there is none whatsoever." However, Dr. J. Spencer Munroe, a New York University professor who injected a laboratory-developed leukosis virus into monkeys in 1963 and found the monkeys developed tumors, says he feels the subject needs more research. Just recently a turkey herpes-type virus has been developed for the control of Marek's disease. It is a live virus. The claims made for it are that the poultry are protected against Marek's disease and that the appearance and numbers of tumors are diminished. However, it does not appear to affect the Rous type of cancers and some of the tumors of the older birds. In addition the leukosis virus may only be masked by the turkey herpes virus so that the tumor response is suppressed, but now the chickens are harboring not only chicken leukosis, but also turkey herpes virus in addition to whatever other cancer viruses they may have. Superimposed on the cancerous viruses are Newcastle disease and coccidiomycosis. However, there is no doubt at all that Rous sarcoma virus is transmissible to the ape. What is man but a fellow primate?

It may be argued that the hydrochloric acid of the stomach will destroy these cancer agents especially when they are also acted upon by the enzymes of the digestive tract. However, as the acidity of the stomach decreases with aging more and more microorganisms are found in the gastric contents from the age of forty upward. The intestinal tract consists of a large bed of absorbing glands and blood vessels. There is no reason to suppose that the intestinal mucosa differentially rejects the tumor agents and their toxic products. Quite the contrary is true. In our experimental animals that were sacrificed after being infected orally by the tumor cultures, the specific tumor agents were found not only in the living cells of the intestine but in the small blood vessels and connective tissue layers. It is well known that the Bittner mammary factor in the mouse is transmitted through the mother mouse's milk. The oral route has been used for immunization with the Sabin attenuated polio strains. There are many diseases that are contracted through ingestion, such as the *Salmonella* group, which contains the typhoid organisms. Incidentally, the *Salmonella* are also carried in the chicken's egg. On occasion, friends have brought me eggs that looked "not right." Often I was able to recover cultures of the *Cryptocides* from them. As one veterinarian said in an interview, "Whatever the hen has is transmitted to the egg as through a sieve."

The question is often asked, "Doesn't cooking destroy the microbes?" I am certain that cooking does destroy many of them. The bacterial stage of the organism dies at 140 degrees Fahrenheit after 15 minutes. When a chicken is broiled it is questionable if that degree of heat is attained around the bones in the fowl. Many Japanese and Chinese dishes are prepared by cooking the chicken for five or six minutes. Also, during preparation, the chickens are washed in the sink where the dishes are washed or placed on the kitchen counter where bread is cut or other raw foods are served. Even if the chicken is prepared away from the usual food counters, if spores of the organism are present in the bird, they are not killed at all by ordinary cooking. They require sterilization on three successive days of autoclaving for twenty minutes under steam pressure of thirty pounds in order to kill them. Also there is no knowledge as yet as to whether cooking detoxifies the toxic material that is present in the infected bird. Since the cancer organisms are transmitted to the egg, the usual cooking of soft boiled or scrambled eggs might not destroy them. The organisms can multiply even under ordinary refrigeration, so stored poultry and eggs may incubate increasing numbers of the agents. Only today a mother called to say that her two-year-old daughter woke up one morning with a swollen eye. It was diagnosed at the University of California at Los Angeles Medical Center as a rhabdomyosarcoma of the connective tissue of the eye. The child is receiving cobalt and chemicals. The surgeons feel that the entire eye and surrounding tissue should be removed. Even with all of this, the mother is promised nothing as to the child's ultimate survival. I asked her what her girl likes to eat. She said, "She just loves soft scambled eggs. I sometimes give her three or four a day."

"This is a very, very serious problem," says Ralph Nader, the consumer crusader. He acknowledges that the evidence for transmissibility of fowl disease to man needs much more research but, he says, "There also isn't any proof to show the disease can't be transmitted. And the research on this has been very recent and not thorough at all." He also said that there are insufficient numbers of inspectors so that "a lot of bad poultry is probably slipping onto your dinner table."

A recent article in the *San Diego Union* was entitled "Leukosis in Every Pot."

> The U.S. Department of Agriculture may be on sound medical ground when it contemplates permitted sale of poultry displaying the evidence of chicken cancer because no definite proof of a link between chicken cancer and human cancer has been proven. Nevertheless it does not help much for the department to assure us that should the tumor be on a drumstick the diseased leg would be ground up for frankfurters. Somehow, it is not even comforting to learn that most poultry, including that we have been eating, is infected with leukosis to some degree. Considering the furor over cyclamates and the Pill, the proposal to relax the existing ban, is, to put it mildly incredible— and inedible.

There are tumor-free poultry flocks in our country. Let's put off a moon shot and clean up the poultry industry whatever the cost.

New York
Academy of Sciences
Meetings in 1969

For three years following the heart attack I suffered in 1962 I was relatively inactive in cancer research. After I had recovered sufficiently I devoted my time to teaching at Calwestern and to community social activities such as the San Diego Symphony, the Children's Adoption Society, the Opera Guild, La Jolla Pen Women and the Vassar Alumnae Association as well as some church activities. I still had my driver-companion who took me around to these meetings. During this period, my friend, Mrs. Betty O., the same one who had brought care packages to me in the hospital, told me the sad news that her husband, Dr. Ralph O., had a malignant tumor of the thymus gland located in the center part of the chest, which contains the heart and large blood vessels as well as the thymus gland. He had suffered a near-fatal car accident a few years previously which necessitated a great deal of blood from the blood bank as well as extensive surgery. He had been in the hospital then for one year. Now he had a lymphoma bigger than a baseball. He was operated on but there was nothing to do since the tumor had grown into all the surrounding tissues and could not be removed. He was informed that cobalt might be helpful but the doctors anticipated that no procedure would really help him. Betty came to see me one day and said, "You know so much about cancer and you're always talking about treating animals. Why don't you help Ralph? There really isn't anyone who can offer him any hope." I was very reluctant to undertake treating him. However, since they were both very dear friends I agreed to try. We used an autogenous vaccine as a nonspecific immune stimulation, mild antibiotics, and diet. It is now ten years since that time and he says that he has remained perfectly well. Dr. O. had a friend who was a physician in San Diego. At this time I collaborated with him and he said several of his patients had excellent results. Also I had worked with a physician in Covina, a member of our church, who also treated several cases, he said, successfully. Dr. O. was so pleased that he asked one of his patients to give me a grant to carry on more of my research. The Fleet Foundation of San Diego then gave me a modest grant for several years. This later formed the nucleus of the present Livingston Fund at the University of San Diego. The gifts from patients and friends have kept the research work going.

In order to receive the grant I had to affiliate with a non-profit group to accept the funds so that the money could be given tax-free. I chose the San Diego Biomedical Group, an association of scientists consisting of physicians, physicists, engineers and college professors. I equipped a laboratory at the Biomedical Institute where I remained for a year working there part-time and at a small office I opened in the neighborhood where I could consult with a few patients on a research basis. Eleanor Jackson came out to visit for a month. During that year I reaffirmed the presence and cultural properties of the *Cryptocides* group and tested all of the strains so that we established an antibiotic profile. The strains were consistent in their sensitivities. In addition, with Dr. William Pincus and my technician, Sherry Boyd, tissue cultures were set up and into these were innoculated various types of filtrates from the cultures. There was no question about the growth-stimulating effects of the filtrates in one phase and in another there was vacuolation and cell destruction similar to the action of well-known oncogenic "viruses." However, the facilities were not adequate there so, when Mrs. Boyd left on maternity leave, I decided to join the University of San Diego as associate professor of biology in residence under Dr. Curt Spanis. Some of the funds I had were used at the University of San Diego to support senior and graduating students as my assistants in furthering the work I was doing. In the summer of 1968 Dr. Jackson came out and stayed three months with us. We had a full-time technician, a medical student, my husband, Dr. A. M. Livingston, and Dr. Gerhard Wolter from State College all working with us in the laboratory at USD. This was a very fruitful time for us. We carried on extensive bacteriological studies with P. *Cryptocides,* which enabled us to characterize the organisms and propose their classifications at the New York Academy of Sciences in 1969. Under our direction Charles Geist, a graduate microbiology student, carried on this work in consultation with Mr. Lester Winters and Mr. John Murphy at the Fourth Avenue Laboratories in San Diego. The chart of the growth characteristics of P. *Cryptocides* is given in the 1969 paper on "The Bacteriology of the Specific Microorganism, the *Cryptocides.*"

About this time aflatoxins were found to cause tumors in fish. Food contaminated with aspergillus produced aflatoxins and these acted as carcinogens in the fish. It seemed to me that since our organisms, the *Cryptocides,* were members of the Actinomycetales group, they should produce actinomycinlike compounds in culture tubes and these substances might be recovered from the urine of advanced cancer patients; and, also, there should be some kind of blood level of these chemicals. We were encouraged in our endeavors by the fact that Dr. Wolter had found a wide deep red-brown ring in the liquid culture at the top of a tube of living organisms that we had given him. He had put it in a dark closet for the summer and in the fall; there was the red-brown material, the same color as some of the known actinomycins. Also, we had collected the urine of terminal patients and found the same coloration.

First we began to collect urines of the dying patients from different hospitals. We went around to the cancer wards at Naval Hospital and collected twenty-four-hour urine specimens from the terminal cancer patients. Large containers with some acid in them were left for the collections. My husband said he was the best collector in town of what nobody wanted. Dr. Wolter then proceeded to extract these urines. The results of urine and culture extractions are reported in our paper of 1969, entitled "Toxic Fractions." This was a pretty malodorous job and Dr. Wolter arose early in the morning to do his extractions at State College in the hope that none of his colleagues would arrive before he had aired out the laboratory. He was successful in making various extractions and isolating a number of different fractions from the urine, some of which resemble actinomycin crystals.

The next step was to find out whether the isolated cultures would produce the same toxic fractions that were extracted from the advanced cancer patients. We obtained large flasks and used the culture media described for the production of actinomycins. These had to be kept in the dark. We made our isolates, harvested a sufficient amount to plant in the large flasks and then waited anxiously for the organisms to grow. It required not less than six days and sometimes twelve for the pale pink to darken and become ruby red. Dr. Wolter then extracted this material and produced crystals which we compared with the material from the patients' urine. This, too, was a dangerous procedure because the extractions done at USD necessitated using an exhaustion hood to prevent the inhalation of toxic fumes. We would work as long as we could and then run outside to sit gasping and panting on the benches along the sidewalk.

Dr. H. B. Woodruff of Merck and Co. in Rahway, New

Jersey, kindly said he would assay our material in comparison with actinomycin for antibiotic activity which would serve as an indicator for the activity of our fractions. We succeeded in getting enough to send to Dr. Woodruff but he reported failure with the first batch. I was sick at heart after so much effort but I decided to ask him what the pH or acidity of the material was. It turned out that there had been a strike at the Merck plant in Rahway and that the material had turned alkaline in storage so all chemical activity had been destroyed. We sent on more fresh material which showed measurable activity comparable to actinomycin. Then Dr. Woodruff grew and extracted more of the chemical material from cultures which we sent him. Since his laboratory is the best in the world for this kind of work we were indeed grateful that he undertook these experiments for us. He then sent us crystals of the material which resembled those Dr. Wolter had obtained in his first studies. Battelle Memorial Institute at Columbus, Ohio, did a few assays for us and assigned the material a tentative formula, $C_{30}H_{38}N_2O_3$. At a later date we sent the Battelle people cultures and material with which they worked for a year. They repeated the work done by Merck, but did no more than confirm the previous studies when our money was exhausted and no further identification of the material was possible. We now have $15,000 worth of crystals in cold storage at State College awaiting further assay.

However, there was one good result occurring from the isolation of the crystals. Dr. Ronald Weider with the consent of Dr. Stanley Weinhouse, at Temple University in Philadelphia, used these materials in a twenty-week pulmonary bioassay test in mice and demonstrated both with the urine and culture extracts a doubling of the number of tumors induced in genetically controlled mice. This is a very expensive procedure so it could be done only once since the work was donated as a gift. These results, too, were reported at the 1969 meeetings.

From November 5-8, 1969, we were able to present our work at the New York Academy of Sciences, section of biological and medical sciences, at the Waldorf Astoria in New York. The conference chairman was Ruth B. Kundsin, Sc.D. of Peter Bent Brigham Hospital, Boston, Massachusetts. The title of the conference was "Unusual Isolates from Clinical Material." Our work from the University of San Diego was presented with Eleanor Jackson acting as chairman of our section, "Microorganisms Associated with Malignancy." I was the first speaker giving Eleanor's and my joint paper on the bacteriology of our specific microorganism and classifying it as Progenitor *Cryptocides,* a member of the Actinomycetales. Just before going to New York with Dr. Curt Spanis, my husband and I went to Los Angeles, where we had engaged the services of an experienced cameraman. We worked an entire day with him and were able to produce an excellent film showing the *Cryptocides* organisms alive in blood specimens of five terminal cancer patients. We showed this film at the meeting. Irene Diller then presented her monumental paper, "Experiments with Mammalian Tumor Isolates." (Bibliography.) Then my husband presented the "Toxic Fractions Obtained from Tumor Isolates and Related Clinical Implications," which was authored by all four of us—the Livingstons, Jackson and Wolter. Dr. Florence Seibert of tuberculin fame, gave her paper on the "Morphological, Biological and Immunological Studies of Isolates from Tumors and Leukemic Bloods." She represented the Veterans Administration Research Laboratory, Bay Pines, Florida. She was followed by Sakae Inoue of Gunma University, Maebashi, Japan, and Marcus Singer, Ph.D., Case Western Reserve University School of Medicine, Cleveland, Ohio who reported an acid-fast organism as the causative agent of cancer in the newt. Then Eleanor read her Rous paper, "Ultraviolet Spectrogramic Microscope Studies of Rous Sarcoma Virus Cultured in Cell-free Medium." Dr. Phyllis Pease of the Medical School, University of Birmingham, England, led the discussion. Other sections at the conference covered mycoplasma, mycobacteria, viruses, and unusual forms of mycotic infections.

The results of our papers were well summarized by the *Diagnosis News* and are reproduced here. We were no longer ridiculed and our work was well received. At USD we received more than five hundred requests from all over the world for reprints of our articles in the *Annals of the New York Academy of Sciences.* At least we feel satisfied that our lifetime of experience and knowledge is now on record in the leading science libraries of the world.

"A microorganism present in perhaps half the population may be responsible for cancer and a variety of diseases of unknown etiology, including scleroderma, arthritis and acute glomerulonephritis," according to several investigators who presented their findings at a conference of the New York Academy of Sciences' conference on microbial isolates.

Summing up about two decades of work, the investigators, from three different institutions, reported that they have found a highly pleomorphic organism in all types of human and animal tumors, in the blood of advanced cancer patients, as well as in patients with certain degenerative and autoimmune disease.

According to their view, the organism may assume a latent form and be inactive as long as the body's defense mechanisms are adequate, but when they are not, disease results. The exact kind of disease depends on the age of the host and its state of resistance.

Some of the other participants at the conference appeared reluctant to accept the idea that a single organism, no matter how pleomorphic, could be so widely implicated. The general feeling at the meeting, however, was summed up by Phyllis E. Pease, D.Sc., of Birmingham University, England. She said the organism or organisms present in cancer patients can no longer be ignored as secondary invaders, but just what they are and what they are doing has not yet been settled. At least they have the potential to cause disease, and the difference between the diseases they can cause may well be quantitative rather than qualitative, she said. Various environmental and genetic factors have also to be considered, she added.

Classification and characterization of the organism was presented by Dr. Virginia Wuerthele-Caspe Livingston, of the University of San Diego. She pointed out that the microorganims of various sorts have been observed and isolated from animal and human tumors for more than a century, and that these have included viruses, bacteria and fungi. But one specific type of highly pleomorphic microorganism has been observed and isolated consistently by her group and others from human and animal tumors "of every obtainable variety" for the past twenty years.

She and her associate, Dr. Eleanor Alexander-Jackson, Ph.D., have now classified it as belonging to the order Actinomycetales, the family Progenitoraceae, and the genus *Cryptocides*.

It is intermittently acid-fast and filterable through filters designed to hold back bacteria. It is sensitive to tetracycline, kanamycin, ampicillin and furacin but occasionally resistant to penicillin, sulfa drugs and mycostatin, Dr. Livingston said.

As for the pleomorphism, it exists as virus-sized bodies of 20 to 70 microns, as elementary bodies of 0.2 micron, and in coccoidal forms of 0.5 micron or larger. The latter are usually gram-positive and resemble common micrococci but are distinguishable by variation in size and the sprouting of filaments or spicules. The organism may also appear in amorphous mycoplasmalike forms, as rods or filaments of varying lengths, and, in older cultures, as spores and hyphoe.

Apparently the organism can invade both cytoplasm and nucleus of host cells in any type of host tissue when body defenses are lowered. In experimental animals it can cause lesions that appear as necrotic abscesses, granulomas, fluid-filled cysts or neoplasms. The type of lesion apparently depends on specific and nonspecific immunocompetence and the age of the host, Dr. Livingston said.

All cancerous bloods she and her associates have examined have revealed these organisms, and she presented a film of untouched blood from a terminal cancer patient in which the parasites were seen in Brownian motion in the red cells. According to Dr. Livingston, they stay inside the cells of patients who are holding their own against the disease, but, in advanced cases, the cells rupture, releasing the organisms.

As a result of her investigations, Dr. Livingston considers malignancy a "neoplastic infection," which depends on the number and virulence of the invading organism, the susceptibility of various organs to it, as well as the natural immunologic components of the host.

Dr. Afton Munk Livingston, also at the University of San Diego, carried this concept further in reporting his work with an extract that has been crystallized from the blood and urine of cancer patients. These crystals are believed to result from the presence of the organism.

He suggested that perhaps half of those in the conference audience carry these organisms which, he said, are "so ancient in origin and ubiquitous in plants and animals that it is virtually impossible to avoid them."

In support of this view, he reported that a study of one hundred random blood samples, taken in the office of a physician who specialized in allergy and immunologic disease, showed that all tumor-bearing patients, in comparison to office personnel used as controls, gave positive cultures for the organism. A number of patients with chronic degenerative disease were also positive. While many patients who had reached a healthy old age were negative, several "tired" young people without apparent disease were positive.

Dr. Livingston reported that a reddish brown material has been extracted from the urine and blood of cancer patients in increasing amounts as they became terminally ill, and that this material has not been found in normal controls. While very little of it has been obtained so far, it appears to be carcinogenic for mice, increasing the incidence of pulmonary tumors. It is hoped that further attempts to isolate and characterize the material will help clarify its role in producing cancer and other diseases.

Isolation of the microorganism and evidence of its disease-producing capability were also reported by Dr.

Irene Corey Diller, Ph.D., of the Institute of Cancer Research in Philadelphia, and Florence B. Seibert, Ph.D., of the Veterans Administration Research Laboratory at Bay Pines, Florida. Dr. Seibert has worked rather closely with Dr. Livingston, but, in independent work over the past twenty years, Dr. Diller has also found the organism consistently in mouse, rat and human malignant tissues and in the blood of tumor-bearing hosts.

She reported that when isolates from mouse tumors were injected intraperitoneally into newborn mice, the tumor incidence was doubled. Furthermore, it was possible to protect the animals against tumors by injecting them with extracts of the same type.

In summing up her work, Dr. Diller reported that the organisms have been cultured from the blood of supposedly normal mice of several strains in proportions comparable to the spontaneous incidence of neoplasm in each particular strain, that mice shown to carry the organisms in their blood as latent passengers prior to the appearance of tumors were the mice that later became tumor-bearing, and that organisms with properties similar to those that were injected were re-isolated from tumors arising in injected mice.

Dr. Seibert reported immunologic studies with the organisms. Labeled antiglobulin, which was specific for the isolate from a human breast, adenocarcinoma induced specific fluorescence in the white blood cells of patients with leukemia and myeloma, indicating an immunologic relationship, she said.

The fluorescence appeared in the same areas of the cytoplasm where other studies have shown the presence of pleomorphic, acid-fast particles similar to the pleomorphic organism in the pure culture isolated from the breast tumor, Dr. Seibert said.

What follows is an excerpt from the latest contribution reporting more recent progress in our work in *Transactions* of the New York Academy of Sciences in May 1972. It is an article written by my husband and myself reporting the recognition of the P. *Cryptocides* organisms in the blood of cancer patients compared with the blood of healthy individuals, of which a summary follows. Examinations by darkfield of fresh blood, and also by brightfield microscope using supravital stains may prove to serve as a diagnostic and prognostic tool in following the course of the cancerous disease in the patient in conjunction with several other microbiological evaluations.

Although the European investigators have not classified the organisms they described as belonging to the Actinimycetales nor have they shown their complete life cycle, nevertheless many of their observations are in agreement with ours. They developed cultural techniques for isolation as well as staining methods after fixation for their recognition. They also employed Seitz filtration and recovered developing forms of the organisms. However, the consistent occurrence of acid-fastness, the marked pleomorphism of the organism, the presence of actinomycinlike crystals in body tissues and in cultures and the development of adaptive stages of the organism such as L-forms, protoplasts, mesosomes, tubules, spheroplasts and tubular structures was not known to them. In addition, their studies lacked the advantage of the electron microscope for the identification of the submicroscopic viruslike forms. Recent definitive biochemical tests such as the cytosine-guanine percentage of the DNA have helped to classify these microbial isolates. Extraction and demonstration of the crystalline material produced by cultures and present in the fluids and tissues of cancerous individuals have been performed. The biological effects have been assayed in preliminary studies with tissue-culture systems and with tumorgenesis in mice. Current efforts are being directed toward characterization of these crystalline substances.

Preparation of Slides for Blood Examination

The patient's finger is immersed in 70 percent alcohol and air dried. A sterile lancet is used to puncture the finger, a small drop of free-flowing blood is placed on a sterile clean slide, and covered with a sterile coverslip. Care is taken that the blood does not flow beyond the edge of the coverslip. Using a small weight for approximately one minute, light pressure is applied to the coverslip to spread and separate the blood cells. This preparation is then examined under darkfield at X 750 and X 1350 magnification. For lightfield examination, the same method is followed and in addition, a small drop of 1 percent aqueous sterile crystal violet, freshly prepared and filtered, is gently applied to the preparation. If the number of organisms in the blood as well as the motility of the various stages are to be evaluated, then the blood is diluted 1:100 with sterile distilled water using a sterile red-blood-cell diluting pipette. The pipette is then thoroughly shaken and a few drops are expelled from the pipette into a sterile Petri dish. A small measured amount of 1 percent aqueous crystal violet is added. This mixture may then be used to flood a blood counting chamber. This method provides a quantitative estimate of the numbers of the organism as well as their motility, which may last as long as fifteen minutes. However, for the usual brightfield examination of the blood with crystal violet, the blood drop is placed directly on the slide and a small amount of crystal violet is added before the coverslip is placed over the preparation and light pressure applied.

Darkfield Examination of Unstained Fresh Blood Preparation
All the illustrations here cited can be found in Appendix 2.

A number of interesting observations may now be made. In the darkfield, pulsating orange bodies in the red cells may be observed. In the background, there are bright dancing forms which appear to be small L-forms of the organism. In severely infected hosts a number of motile rods may be observed (Ill. 3). Spheroplasts and mesosomes both large and small are present. These may have many fine delicately vibrating forms at their periphery. Forms resembling a medusa or an octopus with waving filaments may be present. Organisms may bud from the surface of the red cells and form fine hairlike filaments which resemble the handle of a tennis racquet. There may also be numerous threadlike filaments free in the serum, varying in size, some 10-15 microns in length. These are motile and appear to wind in and out around the red cells. There are also long tubular structures 50 microns or more in length, and about 10 microns in width that are milky white, highly luminescent, containing numerous refractile granules (Ill. 8). The tube in some cases appears to arise from a coalescence of the L-forms or to bud from a spheroplast (Ill. 9). It is transparent since cells can be seen through it. When the tube wall disintegrates the refractile bodies are released in the serum and may enter fresh red cells (Ill. 10). There are also large round milky white forms appearing to be protoplasts about 20-60 microns in diameter which contain granules resembling spheroplasts or mesosomes (Ill. 11). The protoplasts may have budding forms at the periphery and may release rather large vesicular refractile bodies resembling the spheroplasts or mesosomes (Ill. 12). At times, the extruded mesosomes are large enough to be mistaken for red blood cells but they do not have the bluish tinge of red cells seen in dark-field. Rather, minute dancing particles may later appear within them.

In addition, shrunken red cells with a ground-glass appearance spiculated at the periphery may be observed (Ill. 1). We have termed these structures "spent cells" since they appear to be red cells that have been consumed by the parasites. They are lighter and smaller than normal erythrocytes and have a tendency to be pushed to the periphery of the blood drop when it is prepared for examination. Changes in the character of the leukocytes are also apparent. Many leukocytes in the advanced stages of disease appear smudged, inactive and only dimly luminescent whereas normal leukocytes have vigorously active granules and active amoeboid movements. Under some circumstances great numbers of fine spicules occur in the dark field. These are very delicate and appear to arise from minute

L-forms. They are not thrombocytes. At times they appear to shed from the surface of the protoplasts (Ill. 5). Why they should be more numerous at one time than at another is not understood but their appearance may be related to the pH of the blood. Orange crystalline forms of the organism as well as free crystals may also be seen in and around the microbial clusters in the plasma. They apparently arise from the waxy secretions of these mycobacteriumlike organisms. These are the crystals that have been extracted from pure cultures and urines of terminal cancer patients and that have been used for various types of bioassay as previously described.

Brightfield Examination of Supravitally Stained Fresh Blood Preparations

On a blood preparation stained with crystal violet and examined by the brightfield method a clear white light and a magnification of at least X 1000 microbial forms are revealed that are not seen in the darkfield. There are large branching fungal forms that are not luminescent in the darkfield. These fungal forms may extend over a considerable area involving several microscopic fields. Some of these are branching and appear to have conidial or fruiting bodies attached to the branches (Ill. 19). Microcolonies may be clearly seen surrounding individual red cells, and some appear to arise from parasites extruded from the cells. These microcolonies appear to develop into a network of interlacing branching fungal filaments which act as bridges between the red cells and cause them to adhere in clumps (Ill. 15). The number of fungal forms which hold the erythrocytes together or adhere to their surfaces may be directly related to the sedimentation rate. The greater the adherence of the erythrocytes due to the mycelial forms, the more rapid the sedimentation rate. The red cells become separate and free as the number of both intra- and extracellular parasites diminish. The stained preparations in the counting chamber have L-forms, which appear much more numerous than in the darkfield, and occur in clusters, which have marked Brownian movement. These clusters agglutinate and become motionless after ten to fifteen minutes. Introduction of gamma globulin or specific antiserum under the coverslip of the counting chamber causes instant agglutination and cessation of motion. By this method, antibody activity of blood serum can be roughly estimated. Other dyed microbial forms in the brightfield may be compared with those in the darkfield. The vibrating orange bodies in erythrocytes in the darkfield appear as violet bodies in lightfield. The brightly luminous tubules take on a light violet color with deep purple granules.

The same comparison between darkfield and stained brightfield preparations may be drawn by examining blood cultures grown in broth. Hanging drops of cultures sealed with sterile vaseline are preferable to ordinary wet preparations since they are safer to handle and can be preserved for a longer period of time. Conventional staining of slide preparations appears to break up many of the delicate microcolonies and interlacing fungal forms. Wet supravitally stained preparations in hanging drops also indicate the degree of motility of many of the microorganisms. Other dyes have been used which penetrate to some extent but do not provide sufficient contrast. They are Sudan black, saffron yellow, Congo red, May Grünwald, toluidine blue, gentian violet, as well as several others. A further search for useful supravital stains should continue.

In our studies all cancerous patients yielded L-forms as well as other pleomorphic stages on blood culture which, on further cultivation, developed the typical acid-fastness of the Progenitor group as previously described. However, the cancer patient even in the advanced stages of the disease is usually afebrile. Comparable numbers of microorganisms other than the Progenitor group might be expected to produce an acute febrile reaction. There undoubtedly can be a mild or transitory bacteremia in blood due to relatively nonpathogenic bacteria such as some of the diphtheroids. However, with the previously described methods, the great numbers of the Progenitor group as a silent but lethal bloodstream infection may be readily demonstrated, thus justifying the name of the "ancestral hidden killer." Advancing infection of the bloodstream with P. *Cryptocides* is relatively asymptomatic until large numbers of the organisms are present and there is a concomitant breakdown of the immunological and dextoxifying system.

The Orthodox Methods of Cancer Detection and Treatment: Why They Fail

The American Cancer Society has publicized seven danger signals in the hope that persons having any one of them for more than two weeks will consult their physicians. They are: 1. unusual bleeding or discharge; 2. a lump or thickening in the breast or elsewhere; 3. a sore that does not heal; 4. change in bowel or bladder habits; 5. hoarseness or cough; 6. indigestion or difficulty in swallowing; 7. change in a wart or mole. However, the great difficulty is that if the signs lead to a cancer diagnosis, in many cases it is already too late to do very much about eradicating the disease. There are some exceptions such as early diagnosis of breast cancer, skin cancer, and small, well-localized tumors that are readily accessible to surgery. Unfortunately, in many cases by the time the diagnosis is made the cancer is already disseminated. This is neither the fault of the patient nor the doctor but just the nature of the disease. Cancer is truly a "hidden killer." The signs and symptoms of early cancer are often so vague and indefinite that they are frequently overlooked. The person complaining of these signs is often labeled a hypochondriac.

To rely upon the seven signs of cancer is much too simplistic; in fact, even the publicizing of these signs acts as a kind of soporific putting many people to sleep in the thought that if they don't have any of these signs then they do not have cancer. If only that were true. Some people know almost instinctively when something has gone wrong with them. They cannot pinpoint the trouble but they "just don't feel right." They will often describe various vague and fleeting discomforts that have been referred to as "organ recitals." Sometimes they will have one really unusual complaint such as a "funny, itchy feeling," a different kind of headache, a pressure in the rectum that is negative on physical examination, prolonged deep bone or muscle pain, weakness and fatigue, easy bruising, change in body measurement, unexplained anemia and certain skin lesions. They may have small, insignificant looking skin rashes which may resemble scabies or allergic reactions. High or low blood sugar, scleroderma, dermatomysitis and migrating clots in the blood vessels may all be latent signs of the cancer syndrome.

The advice to have two checkups a year is very good and very impractical. There are not enough physicians in the United States nor enough laboratories to carry on these examinations. Just to do periodic chest X-rays in a sense is futile because the early signs of lung cancer are often not detectable by X-ray. By the time they are detectable, it is too late. There is no question that diagnostic X-rays are useful in following the treatment of patients but to rely upon them for the early diagnosis of lung cancer in many cases is useless. Periodic self-examination of the breast may occasionally lead to early detection of breast cancer. Mammography, an X-ray photograph of the breast, and thermography, a test to pick out areas of increased heat, may be useful. No one concedes that these measures will replace actual examination of suspected tissues under the microscope, which is the usual diagnostic procedure. The difficulty is that when diagnosed, 60 percent of the breast cancers have metastasized, and 50 percent are incurable. Leo C. Massopust, Sr., using ordinary photographic equipment plus an infrared filter and film, takes pictures of cancer-suspect breasts. The infrared rays bring out structures two millimeters beneath the skin surface thus revealing the superficial veins of the breast. If the veins are tortuous or engorged, there is suspicion of cancer. In one thousand cases sixty out of sixty-four cancers were identified and there were no false positives. However, whether negative or positive by these results, still the surgical biopsy is the final criterion.

There are a great many other methods of cancer detection that are possible and at times useful, but to perform them on great numbers of patients is not feasible. However, the recent use of isotopes utilizing various dyes and chemicals that have been tagged with radioactive substances has helped to locate tumors of the brain, thyroid, spleen and liver, but some people have questioned whether the isotopes themselves may not be harmful. The use of contrast dyes has pinpointed abnormalities in the kidney and urinary tract. Also contrast-dye lymphography and X-rays of the lymph glands have helped to locate and delineate the extent of lymph-node cancer or metastases. These procedures are useful in guiding the surgeon and enabling him to know how much tissue is cancer-tainted and whether there is enough localization to warrant an attempt at complete excision. Often tremendous extirpations may only debilitate the patient and may not be completely successful in eradication of the disease. The day of taking out the tongue, half the jaw, and all the neck-glands of an eighty-five-year-old lady are mercifully past. It is a painful thought to realize that one in ten patients is subject to unnecessary and futile mutilation.

Over the years, several patients come to mind who presented highly atypical histories and symptoms that eventually led to the diagnosis of cancer. Late one Friday afternoon, a healthy looking, robust woman came to my office. She was the janitress of the local high school. She said she felt fine but a strange thing had happened. The belt on her skirt was too tight yet she had not gained weight. Nothing else bothered her. On examination all that I could find was a slightly doughy feeling in the lower abdomen. Otherwise she appeared in the best of health. On the following day all of her laboratory studies proved to be within normal limits. However, I convinced her that an exploratory laporotomy, a surgical examination of her abdominal cavity, should be done. This was arranged. She was admitted to the hospital on Monday and operated on early Tuesday morning. At surgery it was found that her omentum, an apron of fat over the intestines, and the surfaces of the intestines within the abdominal cavity as well as the peritoneum, or lining, were studded with innumerable small cancers. It was the accumulation of fluid from these multitudinous small tumors that caused the doughy feeling on examination and the tightening of her belt. A small primary tumor was found in the ovary. The ovaries and uterus were removed. In spite of good postoperative care she died of an embolus within three days. Perhaps it was best that she died quickly. This woman neither smoked nor drank. She had regular physical checkups, including Pap smears and blood counts. Obviously, there must be another answer.

Again, on another occasion, a college professor came to the clinic stating that he was feeling very droopy in the afternoon and that, at times, he had a temperature of 101°F. We checked him by every means at our disposal: blood counts, X-rays of lungs and kidneys, urine examinations, various blood chemistries, in other words, the works. He began to lose weight, the fever rose. Finally, a mass was felt in the abdomen. He had a retroperitonaeal sarcoma. It was treated with surgery, radiation and chemicals yet he died in three months. Even if the tumor mass had been detected earlier it is doubtful that the final outcome would have been different.

Today in the university centers there is a new technique called a resonator, which emits sound waves against tissues and gives a diagram or picture of organs and masses in areas that cannot be satisfactorily X-rayed or palpated. Recently this method was used on a patient who we felt might have an abdominal recurrence of a tumor. The report was negative. These are called multiple transverse echograms.

Still on another occasion a woman executive of the San Diego Water Department came in complaining of vague feelings of discomfort in her lower abdomen. Pelvic and rectal examinations, X-rays, all the laboratory tests were negative. She had six more months to complete before reaching full retirement pension. She was advised to take as much vacation and sick leave as she could. Later she worked only a minimum number of hours each day. She was checked regularly every two weeks. She really did not feel any better but she did manage to get through to retirement. Continuing her frequent checkups, she reported that she did not feel any better. One day, some fluid was found in her abdomen. On surgical exploration, a small tumor of the ovary was discovered with widespread metastases to the liver and omentum. It was already too late. Many physicians feel that bizarre symptoms that persist more than a week or two warrant an exploratory procedure of the abdomen in the hope of finding the trouble. Unfortunately even exploration does not mean that the early lesion can be detected.

With all the knowledge that man has acquired, early diagnosis still fails. Too often when the diagnosis is made, the disease is already out of control. The usual treatment of surgery, radiation and chemicals may lead to some prolongation of life but the overall statistics are grim. More sophisticated bioassays are now possible such as the detection of fetoproteins in some cancers such as the liver; changes in hormonal levels, as in lung cancer; and the use of isotopes for the localization and treatment of others.

Another method of treatment is by the use of anticancer drugs. A list of these anticancer drugs now commonly is use are:

1. Hormones: chemical messengers that control the growth and function of various kinds of body cells

2. Analogues, or counterfeits, which destroy cells by mim-

icking essential body elements so that they are incorporated into the cell and thus destroy it

3. Antimetabolites: analogues that block normal cell chemical processes

4. Antimitotics: these prevent cell division

5. Alkylating agents that react with sensitive atomic groupings of the cells' most vital components and behave as poisons

6. Antibiotics: products produced by microorganisms that destroy other microorganisms

7. Radiomimetic compounds that exert radiationlike effects on cell and host chemistry

8. Miscellaneous agents such as antagonistic viruses, microbes, immunity-stimulating agents, various drugs and natural biological and botanical products.

As might be expected, all of the chemotherapeutic agents are similar in their toxicity on rapidly dividing cells of the body such as those of the bone marrow, the gastrointestinal tract and the hair follicles. The unwanted effects are gastrointestinal disturbance such as diarrhea, cramping, bleeding, loss of appetite, loss of hair and reduction of the blood cells produced in the bone marrow. Each agent has its own kind of toxicity. Cytosine arabinoside primarily affects the stomach and intestines, 6-Mercaptopurine can produce jaundice of a peculiar type. Methotrexate is especially toxic to the mouth and produces ulcers of the mucous membranes. The breakdown products of cyclophosphamide appear in the urine where they irritate the bladder and cause bleeding and inflammation. Vincristine, a derivative of the periwinkle plant used to produce the vinca alkaloids, is highly destructive to nerves. Daunomycin, an anticancer antibiotic, is primarily destructive to the bone marrow and in 10 percent of the cases damages the heart muscle. L-asparaginase, an enzyme used to destroy asparagine needed by tumor cells but not by normal cells, causes high fever.

It is argued that it is desirable to induce these harmful effects in the patient in the hope that he might be benefited. According to Dean Burk of the National Cancer Institute only a small percentage of such patients so treated are really helped permanently. The dishonesty of those presenting optimistic highly publicized statistics is shown by the actual facts appended in an accompanying table. The number of patients whose lives are significantly extended is small. The toll to the patient in morbidity such as extreme loss of weight, baldness, ulcerations and weakness is unspeakable. This prolongation of days is not living. It is like pouring a burning concoction into the mouth of a man hanging to the edge of a cliff by his fingernails. He may be roused up enough to hang on fifteen minutes longer; he has not been thrown a lifeline.

Since we know that cancer surgery has only a limited usefulness and that the anticancer agents also cannot be counted on for elimination of the disease, what about radiation therapy? Those interested in radiation should spend some time reading about the natural radiation that constantly bombards us and its effect upon microbial, plant and animal life. The study of radiation is a tremendous one and far beyond the scope of this book. The scientists who produced the bomb that resulted in the destruction of Hiroshima and Nagasaki felt that the great numbers of isotopes that could be produced as a result of their investigations would lead them to understand and control much of the chemistry of life. They also hoped that the isotopes produced might lead to the cure for various kinds of cancer. The first objective has materialized, but the second one has not. Radioisotopes have been used extensively for diagnosis and some for treatment. Suspensions of radioactive gold dust have suppressed tumors. Gold-198 with a half-life of 2.7 days, has been incorporated into nylon thread and sewn through tumors the surgeon was unable to remove. At its peak its energy is equivalent to that of a 400,000-volt X-ray machine. Numerous

Neoplastic Diseases Responding to Chemotherapy

Diagnoses	Polyfunctional Alkylating agents	Antimetabolites	Radioactive isotopes
Leukemia			
Acute, children		6-MP Amethopterin	
Acute, adults		6-MP Amethopterin	
Chronic myelocytic	Myleran ® HN2	6-MP	Phosphorus-32
Chronic lymphatic	Chlorambucil TEM		Phosphorus-32
Hodgkin's disease	Chlorambucil HN2 TEM		
Lymphosarcoma	Chlorambucil HN2 TEM		
Multiple myeloma			Phosphorus-32 Iodine-131
Polycythemia vera	Myleran ® TEM HN2		Phosphorus-32
Carcinoma of lung	HN2 TEM		
Carcinoma of ovary	TEM HN2	5-FU	
Carcinoma of thyroid			Iodine-131
Carcinoma of breast	TEM HN2		
Carcinoma of prostate			
Wilms' tumor	HN2		
Choriocarcinoma, female	HN2	Amethopterin	
Carcinoma of colon		5-FU	
Carcinoma of adrenal			
Carcinoma of testis	Chlorambucil*	Amethopterin*	
Miscellaneous carcinomas and sarcomas	HN2 TEM Chlorambucil Cyclophosphamide		

*Given in combination.

Steroid hormones	Miscellaneous drugs	Results
Adrenal cortical hormones		70% bone marrow improvement; 50% patients live one year or longer.
Adrenal cortical hormones		15-25% improved for several months or longer.
	Demecolcin Urethane Fowler's solution	Patients maintained in good condition during major portion of disease; life occasionally prolonged.
Adrenal cortical hormones		Patients maintained in good condition during major portion of disease; life occasionally prolonged.
Adrenal cortical hormones		Occasional favorable response, but no definite prolongation of life.
Adrenal cortical hormones		Occasional favorable response, but no definite prolongation of life.
Adrenal cortical hormones	Urethane	Symptomatic relief in about 50% of cases, and objective hematological improvement is 15%.
		Prolonged clinical remissions, particularly with P32.
		Brief improvement in about 50% of cases.
		30 to 50% of cases improved for one to three months, sometimes longer.
		Frequently marked improvement in properly selected cases.
Estrogens Androgens Adrenal cortical hormones		20 to 50% improved by hormonal therapy; life may be prolonged in some cases.
Estrogens		80% of cases respond to hormonal therapy; definite prolongation of life.
	Actinomycin D	Temporary regression with 30% pulmonary metastases.
		80% respond, of whom 30% show "permanent" regression.
		15% respond for several months.
	o,p'DDD	Tumor regression and decrease in hyperadrenocorticism in selected cases.
	Actinomycin D*	35% of patients show a favorable and sometimes prolonged response.
Adrenal cortical hormones		In rare instances, favorable responses occur.

isotopes have been combined with carrier materials and implanted into tumors, injected into the blood stream and applied directly to tumor sites. Brilliant and dedicated men have worked assiduously at these manipulations but they have been treating the result of the disease and not its cause.

Many kinds of radiation or X-ray machines have been built to emit various types of deep or superficial rays. Some supervoltage machines can effectively attack sensitive tumors with rifle-bullet accuracy and spare skin and intervening structures. Great care has to be taken that the rays do not injure vital structures. Some radiotherapists feel that supervoltage radiation is far superior to conventional radiation in 70-80 per cent of cancer patients. Those interested in the tabulation of the kinds of equipment used against cancer and described in terms understandable to the layman, are referred to the chapter on radiotherapy in Patrick McGrady's textbook *The Savage Cell*. The five-year survival rates for patients with certain tumors have doubled with the use of modern methods of radiotherapy. These are largely mucous-membrane tumors that are readily accessible. However, the five years inexorably come to an end and then the patient says, "What now?" Is he comforted that he has had his five years? I think not. What about the other 50-60 percent who have not even had five years? The need for long-lasting and effective biological methods is more than apparent, it is imperative.

Many today in the scientific field will admit that cancer and many collagen diseases such as arthritis are due to some unknown antigen, that is, some infectious agent such as a "virus," mycoplasma or bacterium. Since the elusive microbe is postulated today by the scientific world, then identification of the cancer agent and the problem of immunity become all-important. We believe that we have identified this evasive, elusive microorganism to be the Progenitor *Cryptocides* that we have so often described. However, even if the scientific world is not ready to accept this causative agent, still the fact that the cancer process may be infectious is generally accepted. In the light of immunity production or immunity suppression, the various methods of today's cancer treatments must be reevaluated.

The first line of defense to be considered is surgery. Mutilating, destructive surgery sometimes can be effective but generally the patient may be so stressed by the trauma of the procedure that he can never recover. If the lesion is a local one and accessible to surgery, then surgical removal is helpful. Sometimes when the entire tumor cannot be resected removal of part may give the body an opportunity to cooperate in eliminating some of the residual cancer. The same may be said for chemotherapy. At first glance it appears that the cell poisons, although they do not necessarily prolong life, may relieve some of the symptoms in some patients at the cost of the destruction of the regenerative powers of the immune system. Sometimes patients who are immune competent, that is capable of making immune, defensive agents, become incapable of doing so under chemical treatment while others who are not competent may become so. Extensive studies of the ability of the patients to be immunized to various agents should be studied as well as their lymphocytic response to treatment. Since the response is so variable it is impossible for the average physician who administers chemotherapeutic drugs to know exactly what is happening. He is guided by a rule of thumb—the number of white cells circulating in the book as shown by the blood count and the condition of the bone marrow as revealed by bone-marrow biopsy obtained by putting a needle into the bone marrow and asperating some to be analyzed. The immunocompetence of the patient under these conditions remains an unknown factor. Only at the large medical centers under expert supervision can the variations in the level of immunocompetence be evaluated. This is one of the great problems facing the physician today, how to evaluate the ability of the patient to respond to therapy and how to protect him from injury to his immune system.

Radiation, too, has a remarkable ability to suppress immunity. Following a large dose of X-rays over the entire body, animals and humans become susceptible to infections and may die from these in spite of intensive antibiotic therapy. Also, the ability of the body to produce immune-producing cells may be permanently suppressed. A combination of radiation and chemicals such as methotrexate have been used to suppress the ability of the host to reject or discard organ transplants. After therapeutic radiation the normal cell must outgrow the cancer cell for the treatment to be successful. Sometimes there is a rebound after several months when the cancer may grow more rapidly than ever. Whether the tumor becomes resistant to the radiation treatment depends upon the patient rather than on the tumor. Some patients tolerate radiation better than others. The effects of radiation, drugs that inhibit cell division, and hormones that repress inflammatory responses are all vitally concerned in the retention of organs after organ transplants. Also, since the *Cryptocides* may be involved in the initial deterioration of the organ that has been replaced, it may be aroused to further activity by immune suppression in continuing its disease-inducing propensities even to the point that the patient who has received a transplant now becomes more susceptible to cancer. Organ transplants afford a prolongation of life by a number of years to some patients but it is under very abnormal circumstance of immunity suppression that they exist as handicapped individuals subject to future organ rejection and intercurrent infections. The price they pay is the suppression of their immune system and the sure knowledge that their survival time is limited. How much more valuable it would be to track down and treat with prevention the agents that cause the initial disease which destroys the vital organs and necessitates the transplant!

It can be said that orthodox methods of treatment fail more often than they succeed. More than half of the diagnosed cancer patients succumb in spite of all that modern medicine can offer. It is indeed a grim picture. Modern treatment has failed because the knowledge that cancer is an infectious process has been systematically obliterated in this country for many years. Several who have attempted to pursue this line of reasoning have been ruthlessly suppressed if not destroyed. Now the inevitable emergence of the role of microbes and immunity has burst upon the thinking world. The specific microorganism, the *Crypt-ocides*, has been seen for more than two hundred years in its various forms. Many competent scientists have been persecuted because of their beliefs in the infectious nature of cancer. Many helpless individuals have been pushed into their graves by the organized, implacable methods of treatment that have been a matter of prejudice rather than the result of enlightened investigation of treatment that is aimed at the support of the patient in his fight against an invading microbe. How many dying, anemic old men have been strapped to tables under ionizing radiation without any thought that they would be benefited? How many poisonous chemicals have been routinely administered by chemotherapists who are unaware of the underlying loss of immunity in their patients? How many helpless women have had their essential glands removed just to buy a little more time? Indeed, it is a grim picture.

Your Glands and You: What Your Glands Have to Do with Cancer

The advent of the birth-control pill has made almost everyone aware of how hormones affect the human body. The Pill is the result of the manipulation of the hormones of the ovary, the hormonal gland that produces the human egg, which, on fertilization with a sperm derived from the male, causes the initiation of a new life in the human womb or uterus. Some of the ovarian hormones cause the egg to mature and to be pushed out of the ovary into the Fallopian tube where it meets the sperm. The fertilized egg is then implanted in the uterus where life begins. Other hormones of the ovary cause the fertilized egg to be implanted in the uterus and held there. The Pill, a combination of either natural or synthetic hormones, prevents ripening or ovulation with extrusion of the egg. Hence, when sperms are present, there is no egg to be fertilized. These manipulations have the advantage of cutting down drastically on the birth rate. However, the Pill may have helped cause an increase in sexual promiscuity with a tremendous rise in venereal diseases, which are rapidly becoming epidemic in this country. There is a constant search for new antibiotics to counteract the resistance to the known antibiotics by organisms causing venereal disease. Also, there are less known and little publicized other micro-organisms that are transmitted by the sexual act. These are mycoplasma of various kinds. In men they may become very abundant before the appearance of prostatic cancer. In the female they have been implicated in cancer of the cervix, or mouth of the womb. The more sexual partners an individual has, the more likely he is to pick up the little publicized but latently lethal mycoplasma. These have been implicated in sterility, miscarriages and neonatal death. By some of our bac-teriologic studies we have found that at least some of these "mycoplasma" are actually the L-form of the *Cryptocides*. There is an old rumor that has been circulated for years that advises a woman not to marry a man whose wife has died of uterine or genital cancer.

It appears, then, that man harbors microorganisms that are latently lethal, but can exist in a state of latency or even symbiosis, that is, in a tolerant state where the host and the bug mutually respect the other's right to exist and do not interfere markedly in each other's life cycle. Although Koch's postulates are still the standard for determining the pathogenicity of microbes, yet microbes can exist in man without any obvious symptomatolgy. One reason is that the mycoplasma or L-forms not having cell walls do not set up a marked host reaction. The protoplasm of the latent organism can merge with the proto-plasm of the host without too much immunological attention being aimed at the quiet and unobtrusive passengers that are riding along on the life processes of their host. However, these silent fellows can be aroused to fury at times and form an army of invading destructive microbes which can destroy the human host. There are many biological and chemical agents that can awaken the sleeping giants masquerading as peaceful inhabi-tants of a quiet countryside.

This is where a great deal of the controversy in cancer centers as to the role of microbes. Some scientists propose one theory, some another. One proponent feels that the cancer agent is exogenous, or brought in from the outside, another feels that the agent is endogenous and is there all the time but just needs activation. In my opinion, probably both theories are right. From our darkfield studies previously mentioned, we have seen the cancer microbes sitting quietly in the blood with few in numbers in a nonpathogenic state in healthy individuals. Many of these bloods will not yield the *Cryptocides* on cultivation. However, in the sick cancer patient, the *Cryptocides* is present in its full flowering with all of its forms in the invasive state. These bloods yield positive cultures. There are many factors that can lead to the transformation of the nonpathogen to the pathogen, such as aging, a poor genetic immunological system, poor diet and, above all, overexposure to great numbers of these organisms with susceptibility to a foreign strain. The resistance to any disease is relative.

One may well ask, "If these bugs are there all the time, how can they hurt you?" I can only describe what I have observed. My office at San Diego Health Association was on the second floor of the building overlooking a gas station which has since been torn down to make way for Mr. Alessio's big office building, with Mr. A's plush penthouse Victorian restaurant on top. Working in this gas station was an attendant who had a large oozing cancer of the forehead and temple. He did not keep it covered but seemed to enjoy picking at it with his fingers. It annoyed me to have him service my car and I refused to go there. Every day at lunch this man as well as the boss of the station, Mr. Throckmorton, and two other attendants would sit in a group having lunch together. They passed around bags of potato chips, peanuts, cookies and grapes. Eventually the station was torn down. One year later, when we stopped at his new station, we were told that he had died of a rapidly developing cancer of the colon. We asked about his three other employees. The one with cancer of the face was still alive but very ill. The other two had died, one of cancer of the throat and the other of cancer of the stomach. Very possibly the three men who did not have cancer may have had a latent or similar infection that was endogenous but the superinfection with an exogenous, virulent strain led to fulminating disease.

As Theobald Smith, an early biologist, said, "As human beings intent on maintaining man's domination over nature, we may regard parasitism as pathological insofar as it becomes a drain upon human resources but biology teaches us that parasitism is a normal phenomenon." Only recently has the ecological concept of infection had an impact on medical thinking.

> Great fleas have little fleas upon their backs to bite 'em
> And little fleas have lesser fleas and so ad infinitum
> And the great fleas themselves, in turn,
>   have greater fleas to go on
> While these again have greater still,
>   and greater still, and so on.
>   Auguste De Morgan—*A Budget of Paradoxes*

When making observations of blood in the dark-field microscope I am constantly amazed at the enormous numbers of microbes that are present in a tiny droplet of blood from an advanced cancer patient. If there are so many in one droplet, the mind is staggered by the trillions upon trillions that are present in the entire human individual. It is obvious, even to the uninitiated that these blood organisms, as plentiful as the plankton in the sea, are utilizing host materials and excreting great amounts of their own products. There must be a tremendous interplay of the by-products of these microbes upon the host cells. The microbes are living their own lives, secreting enzymes that break down the host's essential proteins for their own use, producing factors that enhance their own growth and protein synthesis, and excreting into the blood of the host large quantities of enzymes, growth factors, hormones, metabolized fats, proteins, carbohydrates, oxidation regulators and numerous metabolic products that may be protective to the microbe but destructive to the host. It is now postulated that microbes affect the lining of large and small blood vessels, even the aorta, where the cholesterol plaques claimed to be the cause of atherosclerosis and hypertension, are shown to be fatty deposits of clusters of microbes that have invaded the wall of the blood vessel. These effects have been amply described in our paper "Mycobacterial Forms in Myocardial Vascular Disease," which has previously been cited.

The actual physical presence of these specific microbes may be far less damaging than their systemic effect upon the host through the interference with the vital processes of life such as protein synthesis, oxidation-reduction systems, and very importantly, the effect upon the endocrine system of the body causing a complete derangement of the hormonal balances that are essential to life.

The plot now thickens when we begin to wonder what effect the products of these microbes, the *Cryptocides,* have upon the hormonal pathways of the human host as well as upon the delicate enzyme systems that are dependent upon them. The human being has a group of endocrine or ductless glands that produce hormones, a Greek word meaning messenger. Substances are produced by these glands that are carried in the bloodstream to distant points where they activate certain end organs or receptors to perform various kinds of functions depending upon the activator and upon the tissue being activated. The chief gland is the pituitary at the base of the brain. As Dr. Harvey Cushing used to say, it acts as the leader of the band. It directs a stimulatory and regulatory action on all the other glands and secretes some substances of its own having to do with water balance. The thyroid gland is situated in the neck and secretes thyroid, which controls oxidation of the cells as well as other metabolic regulatory functions. Almost buried in them are the small parathyroids, which control calcium metabolism. In the stroma of the thyroid glands there are cells that produce calcitonin, which controls the laying down of bone cells. The thymus gland is in the medistinum in the central part of the chest. This gland is very active in the young and has a profound influence on immunity and the production of certain kinds of lymphocytes. The pancreas is near the stomach in the upper part of the abdomen and secretes insulin that is essential to the utilization of sugar and carbohydrates as well as other enzymes which digest protein, fat, and carbohydrates. The adrenals are situated like a cap atop the kidneys and produce steroids and adrenaline. There are some blood hormones such as erythropoietin produced by the kidney itself. The ovaries in the female produce estrogen and progesterone, which regulate ovulation, female characteristics and have to do with the implantation of the fertilized egg in the uterus. In the male, the testes produce male hormones and stimulate the production of spermatozoa. This outline is extremely brief and is intended to serve only as a stimulus to the reader to study more about the endocrine system. What is important, however, is that certain chemicals can have a tremendous effect upon the entire hormonal system. One of these substances is actinomycin produced by several of the actinomyces organisms and probably by many of the Actinomycetales. There is a whole array of chemicals and biologicals produced by this group of microbes, which has been used as antibiotics and antineoplastic agents in some cases.

The actinomycins even in very high dilution of one part in a billion or more may have a profound effect upon the entire business of life. They arrest the maturation of cells, inhibit immune response of many kinds, destroy cell integrity, produce malformation and even death of embryos, inhibit and destroy enzymes of all kinds, and prevent the synthesis of essential proteins, decrease thyroid, estrogen, testosterone, and steroid levels, tear down cells, and poison the host with their toxic products. A reference, the excellent summary by Larry D. Samuels to the action of *Actinomycin and its Effects,* is given in the bibliography. The important thing to remember is that no function of the body is exempt from this toxic material which is produced by these microorganisms belonging to the Actinomycetales.

Not only are the normal functions of the host's hormonal system deranged but there are "false hormones" produced which further throw the body off balance. Dr. Charles Huggins of the University of Chicago won the Nobel Prize in 1966 for demonstrating the effect of the sex hormones on metastatic cancer. He also worked with enzymes and bone physiology. Following his discoveries the practice of castrating men and women to arrest the growth of cancer was initiated. If castration is successful in prolonging life, then adrenalectomy may next be done when the effects of tumor inhibition from the castration have worn off. Adrenalectomy may give one to several more years of life but often none at all or only a few months in the majority of cases. Then the pituitary gland may be removed in the effort to gain more time. Now that there is a simple method to go in through the nose to remove this gland, it has been done fairly frequently for some kinds of cancer. The sex hormones are not usually given for replacement except with hormones from the opposite sex. Adrenal steroids and pituitary gland replacement therapy must then be carried out for the rest of the patient's life or death will result. This hormonal ablation presents a grim picture to say the least.

It is my opinion that the hormonal stimulation of the sex glands, the adrenals and the pituitary are the result of toxic materials or hormonal derangers that upset the balance of the patient's hormones not only by inhibitory effects but by production of pseudo hormones that act on the physiologically controlled, normal glands causing abnormal responses. Also various kinds of cell poisons and inhibitors destroy the efficacy of the lymphocytes to attack the cancer cells. The cancer cells themselves are prevented from reaching maturation by these cell poisons. They are sick cells unable to reach a normal maturity and normal function, wherever they are located and whatever tissue they may be, whether glandular, interstitial, bone or blood.

When I asked Dr. H. B. Woodruff if he knew of anything to destroy the action of these toxins, he said the most important thing was to try to destroy the microbes that were producing the aberrant cell inhibitors and false hormones. In this chapter on treatment, it will be described how this attempt has been made. However, it has been reported that low testosterone levels have been induced in patients with cancer of the prostate by treatment with diethystilbestrol, a synthetic hormone, and amino-glutethimide, a powerful inhibitor of adrenal cortico-steroid biosynthesis, with patient improvement. Furthermore, an immunological mechanism appears to be involved: the inhibition of steroid biosynthesis. By removing the lympholytic effect of corticosteroids, there is produced a marked hyperplasia and increase in the number of circulating lymphocytes which potentiate the immune response. The presence of lymphocytotoxic antibodies have been reported in patients with prostatic cancer. Perhaps this steroid is a "false steroid" and antagonism by the amino-glutethimidine and diethystilbestrol may permit an increase in the production and circulation of normal lymphocytes capable of attacking the cancer cells.

The role of steroids in chronic diseases was demonstrated by Edward Kendall and Philipp Hench in their studies in rheumatology for which they received the Nobel Prize in 1950. At the time of the discovery of the inflammatory blocking power of the steroids it was felt that this would arrest many of the collagen diseases such as rheumatoid arthritis and lupus erythematosis. It is true that the steroids do have an inhibitory effect on these diseases but at the expense of suppressing immunity and permitting the underlying latent infection to continue or to increase in its growth potential. In the beginning of isolation, the steroids were derived from the adrenal glands. However, this was a very expensive procedure which yielded only limited amounts of the material. Now began the era of the application of biological systems to chemical reactions. It was found that a bacterium belonging to the Actinomycetales was able to produce unlimited amounts of steroids from the Mexican yam. This patent is held by Syntex of Mexico. Many microorganisms in the U. S. Patent Office are patented for their ability to produce not only steroids but alkaloids as well. A new book, *Microbial Transformation of Steroids and Alkaloids*, by Iizuka and Naito, has just been released by the University of Tokyo Press. One has only to glance through this book to see the great variety of hormonal and steroidal compounds synthesized by various strains of microorganisms. Microbiologists are constantly on the lookout for new organisms that can perform more tasks in the production of useful compounds.

It is stated that some steroids decrease the numbers of circulating lymphocytes as well as blocking immunocompetence. Perhaps the "false steroids" are really responsible for this action. It has been shown that certain toxic antigens prevent the lymphocyte from maturing and becoming immunocompetent. Leukemia, or an accumulation of large numbers of cells, either lymphocytes or polymorphonuclear leukocytes, may represent a blocking of the pathway to maturity by a toxic agent such as a steroidal or actinomycinlike compound produced by the *Cryptocides*. In a paper "Serum-mediated Protection of Neoplastic Cells from Inhibition by Lymphocytes Immune to their Specific Antigens" by the Hellstroms from the University of Washington Medical School Department of Microbiology attempts to clarify why the lymphocytes which should destroy the tumor cells cannot do so. Perhaps the blocking factor may be related to a protective mechanism directed toward making the *Cryptocides* insusceptible through some biochemical fraction that blocks the immune reaction of the lymphocyte.

There are some tumors that act like glands and produce hormones of internal secretion or endocrine substances. These tumors may be situated in the lung, thymus, pancreas, ovary, thyroid, breast or trachea. In other words, they do not produce endocrine substances from their particular gland stroma but substances from tumors that give rise to Cushing's syndrome, named after the famous endocrinologist from Boston, Dr. Harvey Cushing. W. H. Brown in 1928 reported the first case of Cushing's syndrome associated with carcinoma of the lung. The undifferentiated carcinoma is common to all these patients.

Cushing's syndrome consists of muscle wasting, edema of the extremities, swelling of the face, moon face, mental confusion, polydypsia polyuria and diabetes that has been difficult to control with insulin. There is usually a sudden onset of symptoms of hyperadrenocorticism, which may appear at the same time as the cancer or may precede it by as long as two years. The patients' symptoms may be those of Cushing's syndrome or may be due to the tumor itself such as chest pain, hemoptysis, persistent pneumonitis, shortness of breath. Diabetes was present in all cases and was shown by elevation in fasting blood sugar and sugar in the urine. These aberrant adrenal steroids increase the formation of sugar from amino acids and glycerol and also block insulin with a decrease in the utilization of sugar in the tissues. There is an imbalance of the electrolytes as well as destruction of the kidney tubules. The 17-hydroxycorticoids and 17-ketosteroids were elevated in the urine three to twelve times normal value due to the continued stimulation of the adrenal cortex by the tumor hormone. ACTH was decreased in the pituitary. Methods used to extract the "tumor adrenocorticotropin" are the same as that used to extract ACTH normally. Biologically and physiochemically these two hormones have been indistinguishable and appear to be the same; however final proof is awaited. The secretion of "tumor adrenocototropin" is not suppressed by the high level of circulating corticosteroids. In other words, it is not under the control of the usual host system of controls.

Preparation and Use of Vaccines in Collagen and Neoplastic Diseases

Since it is now generally conceded that cancer and probably many of the collagen diseases are caused by some sort of infectious agent or antigen, the search for these agents is intensified at the present time. Untold amounts of money are being expended in this endeavor. It seems ironical if not humorous to contemplate that these tumor agents are here with us now in the very food we eat, such as infected chickens and eggs, not to mention other infected animal tissues, although probably of less importance. There is also, of course, a certain amount of transmission of the disease from person to person as well as chemical arousal of the latency of the endogenous cancer infection. Our investigations over the years have led me to the conclusion that these agents are members of the Progenitor *Cryptocides* group, a subdivision of the Actinomycetales.

There have been attempts at immunization in the country as well as in Europe using the whole tumor cells as well as various types of extractives. Other intercurrent infections that were fortuitous such as scarlet fever, chicken pox or smallpox occasionally have potentiated an immune response resulting in the disappearance of the cancer. For this reason, researchers for a number of decades have been seeking tumor antagonists not only in the form of antibiotics, which are chemicals secreted by other microorganisms, but through potentiated immunization by the use of other microorganisms. These biologicals are in sharp contrast to the chemotherapeutic agents that seek to destroy the dividing tumor cell regardless of the entailed immune suppression. However, there has been a sturdy, determined group of men both here and in Europe who have attempted to use the causative agent itself as a means of immunization. The difficulty in the United States has been that the scientific world refused to accept the validity of a possible causative agent and discredited the immunization efforts of these early pioneers. Dr. T. J. Glover was forced out of Washington and returned to Toronto an embittered man. Actually it seems that Tom Deaken, a laboratory assistant to Dr. Glover performed most of the experimental work. It appears that Deaken had been inspired by the work of Louis Doyen in Paris who had seen the agent which he thought was causative in his preparations and called them the micrococcus of cancer. Dr. Irene Diller cultured the cancer organism from the blood of mice and used the cultures for immunological procedures as well as for prognostication of which mice would succumb to cancer. The work at the Rutgers Laboratory in Newark preceded the Diller work but was limited to the treatment of a pilot group of chickens with leukosis and to the production of antisera mainly for the study of cross-agglutination and classification. Mostly the Rutgers group was concerned with establishing the validity of the organism, producing pathology with it and classifying it. The later work at the University of San Diego was beamed at trying to discover how the organisms produce toxic materials that are carcinogenic and at identifying the chemical nature of these toxic fractions. My original work in describing the *Cryptocides* as being acid-fast and filterable laid the groundwork for the subsequent theories concerning the nature of so-called viruses such as the Rous tumor agent. Dr. Jackson continued this concept in her Rous studies.

In the State of California the only legal treatments for cancer are surgery, radiation, or chemicals. Any other treatments require that an application for use be filed and approved under Section 505 of the Federal Food, Drug and Cosmetic Act. When such applications are filed, if there is disagreement as to efficacy of the proposed medication, there can be years that pass before such a treatment can be approved. Therefore, such an application opens the door for the absolute regulation of treatment regardless of the harmlessness or lack of toxicity of the product. This is the impasse that has been reached in Laetrile. Since the nitrilosides are contained in food products and are food products themselves, the question of the legality of the restriction of this usage is now under legal challenge.

With the use of vaccines, however, there is a totally different picture. Autogenous vaccines, are prepared and used all over the world in the treatment of chronic, ongoing infections in the sick. Customarily the vaccines are prepared from urine, nasal, throat and bowel secretions as well as from various tissues and other secretions. These are used either for desensitization as for allergic patients or for the building up of immunity in the chronically ill patient who suffers from a failure to produce immune bodies against his chronic infection. This state of nonresponse is called immuno-incompetence.

We use autogenous vaccines in the treatment of many of our patients whether they have cancer or not. In our field of medicine which is allergy and immunology as well as internal medicine, in my opinion patients benefit from these treatments. We do not represent to the cancer patient that the use of autogenous vaccine is proposed for the treatment of cancer but for their underlying failure of immune competence. In many cancer patients we do not use autogenous vaccine at all just as the use of BCG or smallpox vaccine would not be indicated. The use of vaccines must be carefully weighed in the evaluation of the patients' immune status. In some cases the use of vaccines are actually contraindicated. In the seriously ill cancer patient the most important thing is to raise the patient's immunity by the use of fresh, whole blood transfusions from suitable donors, and by the use of antibodies such as gamma globulin. The next most important thing is to treat their chronic underlying infection whatever it may be with suitable antibiotics. The removal of harmful substances from the diet is essential as well as the addition of needed vitamins and nutriments that may be lacking in the seriously ill because of lack of appetite and weight loss and faulty diet. We do not believe that vaccines can cure the cancer patient. It is one of the modalities used for the chronically ill whatever their disease in the effort to restore their resistance to an ongoing, underlying chronic disease. Although the use of various other agents such as autogenous vaccines by the doctors Ruth and John Graham at the Roswell Park Memorial Institute have been widely acclaimed since 1959, it is forbidden by law in California to treat in this manner although the deadly poisons which not only destroy immunity but also produce cancer in their own right are legal. It is now incontrovertible that the cancer disease results in the loss of immunity yet it is treated with radiation which destroys immunity and with drugs which encourage cancerous growth. This is reported in the following abstract and yet the use of the following drugs which produce cancer in experimental animals, are advocated by the FDA and the medical profession as indicated in this abstract:

CARCINOGENICITY STUDIES OF CLINICALLY USED ANTICANCER AGENTS

D. P. Griswold, J. D. Prejean, A. E. Casey, J. H. Weisburger, E. K. Weisburger, H. B. Wood, Jr., and H. L. Falk. Southern Research Institute, Memorial Institute of Pathology and Baptist Medical Center, Birmingham, Alabama 35205, and National Institutes of Health, Bethesda, Maryland 20014.

The carcinogenicity of forty-seven single agents or combinations of agents, mainly anticancer drugs in clinical use, is being studied in Swiss mice and Sprague-Dawley rats of both sexes. All agents were given i. p., usually three times per week for six months, at the maximum tolerated dose (MTD and MTD/2). The MTD was predetermined from forty-five-day tests. Animals were observed for twelve months after the end of treatment or until impending death.

Preliminary findings (among those animals that have come to autopsy) based on gross observations at autopsy and histopathological study of about thirty tissues per animal indicate high incidences of benign and malignant neoplasia following treatment with several drugs, including Melphalan, Chlorambucil, uracil mustard, Natulan, dimethyltriazenoimidazole carboxamide, and 1,3-bis (2-chloroethyl-) and 1-(2-chloroethyl)-3-cyclohexyl-1-nitrosourea. Tumors of several types and at a variety of sites were seen, including adenoma and adenocarcinoma of lungs and breast, lymphosarcoma, leukemia and peritoneal fibrosarcoma.

Only recently I was visitied by an FDA representative from Sacramento who warned me that I could not treat cancer with vaccines. I assured him that I was not treating *cancer* with vaccines but that I am using autogenous vaccines obtained from the patients' own tissues and body fluids to treat an underlying chronic infection. I emphasized the fact that these organisms are not present in cancer alone but also in a host of collagen diseases and in healthy carriers as well, and that the use of vaccines for chronic disease states is an accepted modality in therepeutic medicine. It has never been my intention to state that the use of autogenous vaccines cures cancer. It would be wonderful if it did. However, by giving the patients good nutrition, by helping them fight off chronic infection, and by using any and all accepted modalities that may be helpful, we have tried to assist them in throwing off their diseased condition, whatever is may be. Not to do so would be comparable to refusing a cancer patient an aspirin for a headache on the grounds that the aspirin was being used illegally to treat the cancer.

The production of vaccines from blood cultures is a rather long and tedious procedure. While I was recuperating from my cardiac illness, Eleanor Jackson had visited Dr. W. M. Crofton in Edinburgh, Scotland. He had stated that "there is no cancer the microbial cause of which cannot be grown from and a specific antigen made for its treatment." He claimed he had developed a method of obtaining his specific microbes by direct cultivation of urine obtained with aseptic precautions. The urine was then sent or brought to the laboratory. Crofton recommended using some of the patient's blood to make a blood agar plate on which to streak the urine with a sterile cotton swab. In lieu of the patient's own blood, outdated blood-bank blood has been used combined with the sterile agar in this country. In our laboratory we use the following method for making autogenous vaccines from urine. We use sheep cell blood agar with phenyl-ethyl alcohol, which inhibits the growth of E. Coli, a common contaminant. Either the patient leaves the urine as directed in our laboratory or follows these directions at home.

1. Boil a screw-top bottle and top for twenty minutes. Let it cool. Remove with sterile tongs which have been boiled or disinfected in rubbing alcohol.

2. Take a bath. If a female, take a douche and wash off thoroughly.

3. Using three balls of sterile cotton wash off from front to back three times over the perineum with either Phisohex or some other mild disinfectant such as ST 37. If a male, pull back the foreskin and wash thoroughly three times separately with each of the three cotton balls.

4. Start the urine stream over the toilet bowl and then catch the midstream into the sterile bottle without contaminating it

inside. Be careful to keep the fingers out of the inside of the screwtop cap. Tighten the cap thoroughly to prevent leakage.

When the urine is received in the laboratory it is streaked onto the sterile blood plates using sterile swabs. The plates are then incubated in the usual way. Generally by morning small colonies have formed. When these have been properly identified by allowing the growth to continue for a day or two to be sure that the characteristic colonies are present, then a single colony is studied by Ziehl-Neelsen stain, Kinyoun type, for acid-fastness and the characteristic morphology. Then a single, identified colony is spread on one or two additional plates where they are incubated until sufficient growth has accurred. Stained preparations are again examined. The colonies are then swabbed off into a 2 percent phenol solution and permitted to stand overnight. We then send the phenolized culture to a licensed laboratory where, the next morning or after eight hours, the cultures are diluted to 0.5 percent phenol. It requires about two weeks to complete the sterility tests and to make several dilutions according to government regulations. We do not ship the vaccines out of the state since that is forbidden by law. We prepare only autogenous vaccines tailored for each individual as required by law. The vaccines are made up into 10 million, 100 million and, in later repeated vaccines, as high as 1,000 million or a billion organisms per cubic centimeter. The lowest amount, 10 million organisms per cc, is used as the starting bottle for progressive immunization. Doses are taken every three to five days depending on the reaction. It is wise to start with 0.1 cc by subcutaneous injection of the lowest amount and observe for evidence of redness or soreness at the site of the injection or symptoms of hypersensitivty such as mild fever, malaise, or muscle or joint pains. If there is a mild reaction, the patient waits until it subsides before repeating the same dose or smaller in three to five days by mouth. If there is no reaction, then the dose is increased by 0.1 cc to 0.2 cc and administered first by subcutaneous and then orally in three to five days. The third week, the dose is increased again by 0.1 cc to 0.3 cc subcutaneously and repeated orally again in three to five days. The oral dose is taken in a very small amount of water and held in the mouth for absorption. The vaccine is increased in this manner until twenty drops are taken. Then the next higher number of organisms are started in bottle number two or 100,000 million organisms per cc. The starting dose is 0.1 cc since this solution is ten times as strong as the first one. Again the doses are increased gradually and so on with the other bottles of the vaccines. A vaccine usually lasts six months but if there is quite a change in the character of the organisms under treatment then occasionally it is good to prepare a new vaccine in three months. This method just described is the standard method of preparation of autogenous vaccines and their administration.

The single most important factor in the preparation of vaccines is to rule out common contaminents. The colonies can be entriely confluent in severely infected hosts so that a transplant must be made in order to isolate individual colonies for study. The typical colony has an umbonate (fried egg) shape and may or may not be hemolytic. The colonies may also be wrinkled or smooth, china white or pale tan and even pale pink or orange when grown in the dark. Microbiologists wishing to grow these organisms are referred to our bacteriological papers in the Bibliography. The slides are made by lightly wiping a culture from the plate onto the surface of the glass slide and fixing it with gentle heat. One colony only should be selected and a cross-section should be studied by taking samples from the center outward to the periphery to obtain the different pleomorphic stages. If the material is handled gently the ray formation of the growth will not be broken up. The Kinyoun modification of the Ziehl-Neelsen stain is used since it can be applied in the cold for five minutes and does not require heating. The red dye is washed off with sterile distilled water and the slide is then briefly decolorized with 1 percent hydrochloric acid in 70 percent alcohol. The *Cryptocides* organisms are more sensitive to decolorization by acid-alcohol than the tubercle bacillus. The slide is washed again and the methylene blue counterstain is used briefly and washed off. After the slide is air-dried it is ready for examination under the light microscope at not less than X 800 with oil immersion. If slides are prepared from tissue impression smears of tumors, the same procedure is followed but also Jackson's triple stain may be applied to duplicate slides in order to differentiate the non-acid-fast forms from common contaminants. At times, the *Cryptocides* organism is not acid-fast in some stages of its growth.

Usually the organism isolates out in the coccal form which has led many investigators to believe they are dealing with a staphylococcus. However, the cocci will be both acid-fast and non-acid-fast and will vary greatly in shape from the very small to the large glodoidal or sac forms which often stain blue and appear to be spilling out the red acid-fast cocci much as marbles out of a bag. In addition, the cocci appear to split longitudinally into small rods. The cocci, after a period of time, have small filaments sprouting from them which turn into rods that are red or acid-fast. If the culture is not mutilated by rough handling, often the large tubular forms can be seen which are observed by darkfield microscope in fresh blood. These are very delicate and disrupt easily. The ray formation may also be apparent but the sheath is extremely diaphanous and is destroyed often in the staining process. Sometimes the cancer organism can isolate out primarily as a rod or even as a branching hyphal form. At other times clublike bodies are seen which are blue in color and contain the acid-fast bodies within them. It is very important to study a number of the colonies on the plates and to be sure that the various transitional forms of the organism can be seen in one isolated colony. Only then may the organism be grown in sufficient amount to harvest for the vaccine. All of this work requires careful examination and experience to be sure of the growth pattern and morphology of the *Cryptocides.*

The organisms isolated from the urine cultures have been classified under various names such as staphylococcus epidermidis and enterococcus fecalis, in other words, common organisms found on the skin and in the bowel. However, by careful sterile methods microorganisms are found to be growing in the urine in great abundance. Microbiologists are still debating the nature and classification of these organisms. A recent paper (which appeared in *Transactions* of the *New York Academy of Sciences*) by Dr. Florence Seibert, a famous microbiologist well-known for her work with tuberculin, claims that these isolates from her material which yield certain supposedly well-known microorganisms are not the standard well-recognized types at all but the acid-fast organisms which we have classified as the *Cryptocides*. Microbiologists who examine our urine cultures state that we have a variety of organisms in our urine vaccines. What we do know is that these organisms occur in large numbers and are often hemolytic, destructive of blood. On acid-fast stains they appear to resemble one another but what they really are is still unsettled. Very possibly urine cultures contain a mixture of whatever microbes that happen to filter through the kidneys from distant body foci. We use them only as a nonspecific immune booster in chronic disease.

There are a number of identifying biochemical tests that can be applied but these are too time-consuming and expensive for a routine laboratory. It is hoped in the future that some simple test may be devised for a quick method for identification, thus eliminating the necessity for study of individual colonies. In the dying patient, a few drops of blood taken from the antecubital vein of the arm will grow out furiously on direct plating on the solid blood plates. Usually, isolation from blood is done by placing only a few drops of blood, about five, in the bottom of a trypticase soy-broth tube, and incubating. The organisms can be readily recognized either in hanging drops of the living cultures or by appropriate staining. The organisms grow up the side of the tube forming a lacy pattern and then produce a pellicle or doily on the surface. These are usually motile rods. This is a good stage from which to make a vaccine. As the pellicle ages it has a tendency to drop into the tube again and the spore stages are then formed. The spores cannot be used for vaccines as it is almost impossible to kill them. The liquid cultures will often transfer to solid media plates. Dr. Jackson has developed a sensitive peptone broth for primary isolation which is useful. It can be obtained from the Colorado Serum Company in Denver, Colorado. Dr. Diller's paper gives the various methods of isolation using the technique of Von Brehmer, Glover, Seibert and others. We have also used synthetic broth media for primary isolation but these proved to be too toxic on animal experimentation.

There are several other ways of making primary isolations of the *Cryptocides*. Sterilely obtained tumor tissue fresh from the operating room can be placed into liquid media and later transferred to solid blood plates. Some people have ground up the tumors, filtered them and then cultured them. This is difficult because of the problem of maintaining sterility. These methods led to the recovery of the specific microorganism, the *Cryptocides*. Still others have made various extractives of the tumors with alcohol, acetone or other solvents and used these for the vaccine. Another method is to grow the organism from one of its favored spots, the roots of infected teeth or tonsils. However, the mouth contaminants must be eliminated. Still another way is to dilute the patient's blood with equal parts of distilled water in order to disrupt the red cells wherein the parasites are contained as well as in the serum. The tubes are lightly boiled over an open flame two or three times and then incubated for eight to twelve days. Intervening examination of the blood will reveal the rate of growth. When the growth is abundant, usually in ten to twelve days, the blood can be filtered to remove larger particles, then formalinized, standardized and tested for viability. This method may have some advantages over the whole-cell antigens obtained by the Crofton method because the whole-blood cultures will also contain toxins and antitoxins as well as many of the minute forms which do not grow out on artificial media. This is the German method.

This is an area where a large grant would be most useful to determine the way to prepare the most effective vaccine by animal protection studies against inoculation of specific tumor agents. The practice of transplanting is now less popular than it was since often the survival of these tumors has to do with tissue rejection rather than with any action against the cell-contained tumor agent. Often the mouse host of the transplanted tumor is only the carrier of the tissue and becomes involved systemically late in the disease. Since the tumor agents can now be isolated directly it is more appropriate to use the causative agent in a suitable host. The growth curve of the *Cryptocides* could be plotted and the point of greatest activity as determined by the production of nucleic acids determined. The chemical nature of the compounds elicited by their growth could be characterized and compared with compounds from other organisms belonging to the Actinomycetales. Skin test studies for delayed hypersensitivity in the human host should be done with material similar to the tuberculin test for tuberculosis. Dr. Florence Seibert has proposed this method for cancer detection but no one has followed up on it. Routine blood and urine cultures could be done to determine which individuals are susceptible to cancer formation much in the way that Dr. Diller has done with her mice. Perhaps repeated oral immunization of the entire population might prove preventive. Also by this same method we could clean up our poultry and livestock upon which we depend for subsistence. It is even possible that the immunized animals might transfer some of their immunity to the ultimate consumer, the top of the food chain, us.

Vaccines are now used routinely for the prevention of many diseases such as smallpox, typhoid fever, tetanus, measles, diphtheria, whooping cough, cholera, and polio to name the most common. Various types of immunizing agents are used ranging from attenuated viruses such as the Sabin strains of the polio group, the adapted cowpox for smallpox, the killed bacteria as in typhoid, and the toxoid of tetanus. In polio it was found that the living attenuated strains were more immunogenic than the killed organisms. The polio strains were weakened to the point that they could not produce polio in the person taking the Sabin Sip but strong enough to induce immunity in the Peyer's patches, the islands of immunity producing cells in the walls of the intestinal tract. In other words, the human host was colonized by the weakened organisms which induced immunity to fight off the virulent strains. Live colonization also means that anyone in personal contact with the person who has ingested the living strain can also be colonized by association. However, there may be side effects that are not necessarily predictable. There is a physician who is a rheumatologist in a small town who states that after the administration of the Sabin Sip in his town many of the rheumatoid arthritis patients had serious flareups apparently from an immunological drain that may have triggered their latent infection.

However, there can be far graver results from mass immunization than the activation of reservoirs of latent diseases in the general population. Witness the Salk vaccine fiasco previously discussed. With routine, and, in some cases, mandatory mass vaccination in some countries the potential for catastrophic disaster exists. Where live vaccines are used as in the Salk and Sabin polio vaccines, an undetected infectious agent can be present in the animal culture cells used to prepare the living vaccines. I might hasten to add that this is not the case with the autogenous vaccines which we are using since they are thoroughly killed and carefully tested for viability. However, the accidental infection of multitudes of people here and all over the world has already happened once. Millions of people have been injected with a monkey virus, Simian Virus 40, which was found in 1961 to be contaminating polio and adenovirus vaccines. The virus causes cancer in hamsters and severe kidney damage in other laboratory animals; no one yet knows the extent of harm it may do in man. After the summer of 1961 this situation was corrected but in the years previous to 1961 millions of people were infected with SV-40.

In June 1960 doctors Maurice Hilleman and B. H. Sweet of the Merck Institute for Therapeutic Research demonstrated that recruits given a Sabin vaccine produced antibodies against the SV-40 contaminants. In September 1961 Dr. C. W. Hiatt of the National Institute of Health reported that during the summer he had succeeded in deactivating not only SV-40 but four other simian-virus particles as well by a simple procedure. He had added trace amounts of a dye, toluidine blue, to the vaccine and pumped it through a coil surrounded by a bright white light. This destroyed SV particles numbered 1, 15, 12 and 40. Other particles survived but their effect on the human race no one knows. The vaccines in the Soviet Union and Cuba were decontaminated later. Now the vaccines are produced from healthy human cells. There is a great deal of infighting at the present time as to who was responsible for these recent fiascos. The Division of Biologics Standards had been established after the Salk catastrophe but the new disaster still occurred. In addition, great quantities of ineffective influenza vaccines are claimed to have been released by the DBS.

Since cancer-producing agents are noted for long periods of latency and since SV-40 causes cancer and kidney lesions in hamsters, as well as leukemia in other experimental animals, no one yet knows what it may do in man. That it can do something is fairly certain from recent reports in the *New England Journal of Medicine,* February 24, 1972, Volume 286, number 8, entitled, "Virus related to SV-40 in Patients with Progressive Multifocal Leukoencephalopathy" by Weiner, Herndon, Narayanm, Johnson, Shah, Rubinstein, Preziosi and Conley. This disease is characterized by the loss of the myelin covering of the brain and is associated with an underlying disorder of the reticulo-endothelial system in which there is immunological impairment similar to that in leukemia, cancer, tuberculosis, lupus erythematosis and immunosuppression for renal transplantation. Death usually follows in the course of three to six months. Inclusion bodies are seen.

The abstract of the article states, "Virus related to Simian Virus 40 (SV 40) was isolated from brains of two patients with progressive leukoencephalopathy, a human demyelinating disease. Virus was grown out in cell cultures of primary African green-monkey kidney inoculated with cultures derived from patients' brains. Electron microscopy showed viruslike particles resembling papovaviruses in the brain of one patient and in monkey-kidney cell cultures infected with both virus isolates. Immunologic studies using florescent and neutralizing antibodies indicated a close relation between the isolated viruses and SV-40."

Governments and their agencies are brought together under the law to perform what no one individual either morally or eithically would think of doing. Why must man in the mass be less moral than individual man? Lynchings, wars, power struggles, medical irresponsibility, disregard of poverty, failure to treat each man as a brother, characterize not only individual governments in small communities but nations as a whole led by the sinister men who seek to dominate the bodies, minds, spirits and souls of their fellow men for their own aggrandizement. In the end, it is only the Angel of Death who reaps the harvest of the power struggle.

Care of the Patient

When a patient comes to a physician for advice and help the physician is obligated to give unreservedly to that patient the benefit of his knowledge and skill. Especially when a desperately ill patient seeks help because he knows that his life is endangered by a relentless disease then the physician must give all that he has to give in a spirit of love and devotion. The patient must feel that he is treated with respect, deep concern and a desire on the part of the physician to do all that can be done to alleviate his pain, and to improve his condition, by applying all the information and skills that are available.

When a new patient enters the office it is necessary to become receptive to the needs of that individual. This is accomplished by spending sufficient time with him in a personal interview, in order to learn as much about him as possible. There must be an orderly, analytical, objective, but sympathetic communication established. If the physician is sensitive, before the patient speaks a word, he can identify himself with that patient in a spirit of empathy. Immediately the physician becomes a photographic plate in which hundreds of small impressions produce a picture. How does the patient walk? Is he in pain? Is he depressed? Is he putting on a brave front? What is his general appearance, the color of his skin, his eyeballs, the texture of his hair, the way he handles his body, his odor, his attitude in coming here? All these small things register. The attitude of the member of the family and/or close friend who comes with him, their concern, their insight into his condition, their willingness to cooperate, all add details to the picture. Often the interview will start with a burst of information on the part of the family or patient. It is very important to let them say what they have to say first, before then beginning the orderly probing into the background and history of the patient.

Everyone who has gone to a doctor knows about giving a history. It is good to have the patient write out his historical record before the interview starts. This saves time and helps the doctor fill out essential points. The family background is very important. Many diseases such as diabetes, cancer and mental illness are hereditary. The kind of home he had as a child, his interests and education, his diet including favorite foods, the success or failure of his marriage, the number of children he has and the kinds of friends he has, his occupation, his sense of fulfillment in life, his religious attitudes, all are important. Does he want to live? Has he a death wish? Will he extend himself to regain his health? Is he motivated?

The past history is critical. What took place before he discovered he had cancer? A serious accident? A life crisis? A crash diet? A series of increasing stresses? Chronic disease, fatigue, poor diet? How did the disease start? Early symptoms? When did he first see a doctor? What was done? Surgery, radiation, chemicals? How is he now? What treatment is he receiving? The probing proceeds little by little. Most important, the pathological report and all the medical records must be made available for evaluation.

The patient is then examined and careful notes are taken of

the course of the disease. What are its present manifestations? What reparative surgery has been done? What ablative surgery? Breast amputation, resection of nodes, colostomy, removal of vital organs, orchidectomy, oophorectomy, adrenalectomy, hypophysectomy? Evidences of metastases are sought in nodes, skin, bone, liver, lung, unhealing ulcers on the chest wall, interference with circulation, swelling, localized areas of pain, poor teeth, coated tongue, foul breath, limitation of motion, fluid in lungs or abdomen. The probing fingers and mind of the physician go on and on seeking answers, evaluating the present situation and condition of the patient in respect to what can be done to correct, ameliorate or merely to palliate the disease.

Every conventional method of diagnosis must be employed including blood counts, urine analyses, blood chemistries, determination of electrolyte balance, the kinds, types and amounts of circulating antibodies, thyroid function, blood proteins, steroid levels, various tests for collagen diseases. Radioisotope scans of liver, brain, thyroid are ordered if indicated as well as mammography, photography, or thermography for the determination of breast pathology, multiple transverse echograms for delineating the presence of masses in the abdomen; contrast dye studies of the gallbladder, lymphatics or kidneys, diagnostic X-rays as needed. All of these modalities must be employed in order to ascertain what methods of treatment might be helpful. The patient should be referred to specialists in various fields of competence. The previous or referring physicians should be contacted. A careful evaluation is made of what can or must be done.

Although immunotherapy is the hope of the future for the cure of cancer to supplant the present-day methods of treatment such as surgery, radiation and chemical blockers of cell replication, yet the proven methods must be given the opportunity to make their contribution. Old diagnostic techniques must be employed because they represent the accumulation of knowledge up to the present time. Perhaps there will be a simple serological test for the detection of cancer such as the

Wassermann for syphilis. Perhaps a single cure such as penicillin for venereal diseases. Perhaps an immunological program will be the answer. Unfortunately that time has not yet arrived. However, the many failures of conventional cancer treatment have spurred the entire scientific world on to a search for better methods. When the patient comes to our office, we employ the following procedures.

1. We obtain a clean-catch urine from the patient. This urine is cultured and the organisms are isolated and used to prepare an autogenous vaccine. The numbers and kinds of bacterial colonies are very important, whether hemolytic or confluent, increasing or decreasing in numbers after treatment.

2. The microbial isolates are used to perform antibiotic sensitivity tests to determine which antibiotics might help the patient.

3. A urine culture is made twice a week in the beginning in order to determine the numbers and characteristics of the colonies and whether the antibiotics that have been selected are still effective or whether they have developed bacterial resistance, in which case a new antibiotic must be chosen.

4. Darkfield and brightfield microscope examinations with supravital staining of a fresh blood droplet is done on every visit. As described previously this technique can be extremely helpful. The advanced cancer patient has many forms in his blood in vast numbers due to the loss of immunity. Only time and experience can teach an investigator how to read these slides but almost anyone with some bacteriological experience can learn to do this procedure with practice. Von Brehmer, Fonti, Villequez, Mori, Freiberg, Enderlein all employed the examination of fresh blood by darkfield as a method of following the stage of immunity of the patient. With our present knowledge of L-forms, mesosomes, spheroplasts, protoplasts, and tubular bodies and spicules the evolutionary forms of the *Cryptocides* is better understood.

Treatment

1. We eliminate all poultry products from the diet, even eggs in baking because some toxic fractions may survive heating; all sugars, since many organisms live in the intestinal tract and multiply in great numbers during fermentation of sugars and starches such as are present in candy, cake, ice cream, pastries, carbonated drinks, all of which may "feed the bugs." Overpurified foods such as white flour are also forbidden, since recent research has shown them to be lacking in good nutritive elements.

2. Smoking is stopped because tobacco is a known carcinogen. Alcohol is also not allowed because the detoxification of alcohol puts a tremendous strain upon the liver.

3. A suitable diet will be listed below.

4. We recommend fresh whole-blood transfusion from a young, healthy member of the family. No blood-bank blood. Stored blood loses much of its efficacy in many ways such as oxygen-carrying power, enzyme activity, antibodies, also if there are infectious agents in the blood, such as *Cryptocides*, these may multiply during storage, etc. If the patient is not too acutely ill transfusion may not be necessary. Often sufficient amounts of good fresh blood will cause a tremendous upswing in the sense of well-being.

5. We use gamma globulin largely of placental origin. Parke, Davis and Co. is a good brand. Where transfusions are not given, gamma globulin can be given in a large loading dose as in the acute leukemic, sarcoid or lymphomatous patient. If a loading dose is not given, then 5 cc can be given two or three times a week.

6. Splenic extract, called Pantigen made by the Pasadena Laboratories in Pasadena is given, 2-5 cc two or three times a week. This material is nonallergenic and serves to increase the white blood count. Also spleen is known to enhance immuno-

genic systems. Fresh spleen has been observed to cause remission in the cancerous patient. The intact spleen acts to cleanse the blood by removing the intracellular parasites that circulate in the red cells. In Hodgkin's disease often the spleen becomes secondarily infected and is cut out for the same reasons that chronically diseased tonsils are removed.

7. For four days donnagel with neomycin is administered in the attempt to diminish the numbers of *Cryptocides* if present in the intestinal tract. Then fresh yogurt such as the Continental brand is used or Lactinex or Bacid tablets which contain the living lactobacilli.

8. A tuberculin test is administered to see whether the patient has immunity to the tubercle bacillus. Often patients will tell you that they have been positive in the past. A recent test showing them to be negative indicates a change in their immune state. If they are negative BCG can be given in a single dose intracutaneously. The reaction is carefully watched as it may serve as a guide for further treatment with vaccines of various kinds. Sometimes a markedly positive tuberculin test may light up a small tumor and cause it to swell or discharge. The patient is retested in three months by purified protein derivative (PPD). If negative the BCG may be repeated.

9. Small increasing dosages of nonspecific vaccines are used. These can consist of material from teeth or tonsils, or Staphylococcus Phage Lysate (SPL) made by Delmont Laboratories in Swarthmore, Pennsylvania, or Mixed Vaccines for Respiratory Infections (MVRI). Many physicians both here and abroad like SPL very much as an immune system arouser. Other immunological tests with other antigens are best performed in a hospital under supervision. They are interesting from a research point of view.

10. B-complex, B-12, liver, multiple vitamins are often given as indicated.

11. When the autogenous vaccine is ready it is given as previously described. Reactions must be watched for very carefully so that the patient is not overdosed. Overdosing might, though rarely, result in an immunological breakdown, as is true of any antigenic material.

12. The antibiotic program is extremely important. If the right antibiotic is selected and administered in large doses, the tumors themselves can diminish in size. Some investigators claim this effect is due to concomitant nonspecific infection of the tumor mass, which responds to the antibiotic. We do not use nephrotoxic antibiotics. Frequently, we use bicillin or penicillin G or ampicillin in large doses for a very long period, even six months as advised by Dr. H. B. Woodruff. One patient in a remission from inoperable sarcoma of the neck has been on erythromycin for four and one half years. His disease is entirely under control and he works daily as a longshoreman. Ampicillin by mouth is very useful. Lincomycin and cephalothin are useful for short-term administration. Mendelamine is a good medication to give with the other antibiotics. The furadantins can also be helpful. Each case must be carefully evaluated by blood examination and by urine culture followed by frequent sensitivity tests. It must be borne in mind that the kidneys act as a sieve not only in excreting metabolic waste products but in filtering out bacteria which are in the blood stream from tumors or from established colonies in the intestinal tract or prostate. Sometimes the urinary tract supplies many of these organisms due to direct infection. This can also be determined.

13. As soon as the autogenous vaccines are ready they are started as previously described.

Adjuvants

We give a 5-10 percent solution of magnesium chloride to acidify the blood and urine since a state of imbalance toward the alkaline side is known to exist in tumor patients. One or two teaspoons four times a day are given in a little water. Hydrochloric acid in various forms can also be given. The acidity of the urine is checked frequently with Nitrazine paper. We are hoping soon to be able to check the pH of blood directly. The patient is advised to keep the urine below pH 6, pH 5 if possible. Sea salt is used in food instead of table salt as the sea salt contains trace minerals. We also prescribe trace minerals and especially organic iodine such as is contained in kelp since iodine is essential in the metabolism of thyroid, the oxidative hormone. Additional thyroid is also given wherever tolerated. The suppressive hormones are continued in courses where they have been shown to be helpful such as stilbestrol in male prostatic disease, and nonmasculinizing androgens in women. However, their use is often limited as to long continuing efficacy. Steroids are used very cautiously to suppress the swelling of tumors during therapy. Probably dexamethasone is the least inhibitory in its action on immunity. These are given in short course or in small amounts. Many other supportive measures are given as indicated.

Diet

We have attempted to establish a rational program in respect to vitamin intake. We are aware that many natural substances have been found to be curative before their exact chemical nature and applicability were known. This applies to vitamin C in scurvy, vitamin B in pellagra and schizophrenia, vitamin E in fertility and oxidative processes, vitamin D in rickets, liver fractions in pernicious anemia and so on. The nitrilosides may also fall into this category.

Vitamin Schedule for a Healthful Diet

Dosages should be obtained from nutritional experts.

VITAMIN A

VITAMIN B
  Crude yeast
  Pantothenic Acid
  Riboflavin
  Niacinamide
  B-complex injectable
  B-12 injectable

VITAMIN C

VITAMIN D

VITAMIN E

BIOFLAVINOIDS

ENZYMES

Mineral supplements such as those put out by Plus Products, which contain calcium, magnesium and phosphorus. Include three tablespoons of vegetable oils daily such as soy, sunflower, corn, rednut or sesame.

The diet should contain suitable amounts of protein, carbohydrates, and fats, both saturated and unsaturated, as well as liberal amounts of raw fruits and vegetables.

Sample Diet

Breakfast: Whole grain unprocessed cereal. Whole orange. Fresh fruit such as melon, papaya, pineapple, etc. Whole unsalted, raw nuts such as walnuts, almonds, cashews, etc.

Midmorning: Glass of fresh, raw carrot or other vegetable juice.

Lunch: Whole-grain bread, fresh butter, unfermented cheeses, fresh vegetable soup, fresh fruit, another orange.

Midafternoon: Whole grain bread and honey. Raw vegetable juice, fresh fruit.

Dinner: Portion of well-cooked good-quality meat or fish. Baked potato with skin, brown rice, kasha (buckwheat), whole-grain noodles or macaroni. Large raw salad of many kinds of vegetables especially grated beets two or three times a day. Spinach, comfrey, lettuce, dandelions, watercress, bean shoots, jicama, etc. Raw fruit for dessert.

Bedtime: Whole grain bread, butter and honey or whole grain hot cereal. Fresh fruit or vegetable juice, nuts, raisins, apricots, figs, dates, apples, freely whenever desired. Viable unsweetened yogurt at any or with all of the meals.

Buttermilk, 2 glasses per day.

Avoid all chemicals, cleaning solutions, solvents such as paint removers and insect sprays.

One patient recently had a severe setback shampooing her living-room rug with a cleanser that contained a benzene solvent. The benzene derivatives as well as all toxic materials are detoxified in the liver. A liver already damaged by disease cannot sustain further stress.

The benefits of using large quantities of milk in the diets of cancer patients is debatable. Adelle Davis recommends it. The Laetrile diet forbids it. Many investigators wonder how much growth hormone intended for the young calf is present in the milk. When the ovaries, adrenals and pituitary glands are removed to prevent stimulation of cell growth in breast tumors, the possibility of adding a growth stimulating hormone from milk must be considered, especially when cattle are fed diethyl-stilbestrol, a synthetic hormone. There appears to be no reliable data available at this time as to the growth stimulating hormones in milk and whether there may be a stimulatory effect on normal human growth or an added stimulation of abnormal cells such as is present in tumors.

Disputed Methods of Treatment

For the sake of completeness I am mentioning some disputed methods of treatment. Since I have always made it a policy to treat patients only with medications that are legal in the United States I have no direct experience with materials such as Krebiozen, or Carcalon, as it is now called. I have always had a great deal of respect for Dr. Andrew Ivy and particularly since he has practically laid his life on the line in defense of his theories. Originally Krebiozen was prepared by Dr. Stevan Durovic on the basis of the hypothesis that the reticulo-endothelial system could be caused to secrete an antiblastic or growth-regulating substance into the bloodstream in larger than normal amounts and that the substance could be extracted from the bloodstream by an organic solvent. An extract of *Actinomyces bovis* is used to stimulate the RES. It causes a granulomatous tumor in cattle called lumpy jaw. It is believed that an anablastic material would be secreted to oppose the proliferation of the Actinomyces. Horses were immunized and serum extracted and purified. Many claims as to its efficacy have been made. I have one friend who had a mammary cancer proven by biopsy who took only Krebiozen. It is now eight years and she says she has no evidence of cancer at the present time. I have seen some evidence in treated cases that the tumor was slowed down. I think the basic theory is good just as Leonell Strong's search for the liver factor which suppresses the neoplastic process in mice for several generations could prove to be very valuable. I think these dedicated men should be supported and encouraged as certainly their biological approach is far more reasonable than the continued search for deadly chemicals which destroy instead of enhancing the immune system.

The recent use of *Bacillus* Calmette-Guerin, an attenuated tubercle bacillus, called BCG in the treatment of some kinds of cancer is in a sense a vindication of Dr. Ivy's work. BCG has been found to halve the death rate by leukemia in children in Quebec, Canada. A three-year study has been shown that children under fifteen in the Province of Quebec who were vaccinated against tuberculosis appeared to have only half the death rate from leukemia as children who were not vaccinated. The BCG administration in areas with a high incidence of endemic leprosy is under investigation as providing immunologic protection against the leprous infection. BCG vaccine has recently been reported to trigger remission in melanoma, an almost universally fatal cancer of the skin and internal organs often starting from a black mole. There was a rising titer of antibody and temporary tumor regression in four out of eight patients and a complete regression in a fifth who is free of disease at two and a half years' follow-up. From the last Science Writer Seminar in Clearwater, Florida, 1972, comes the report that BCG is used to fight mammary and lung cancer. In another report twenty-nine patients with malignant melanoma or sarcoma that were treated with BCG experienced reduction in their tumors. Some regressions have lasted up to four years and four patients are now free of disease. In some animal experiments the BCG vaccine has caused cancers to regress or disappear in two-thirds of cases. Only cancer patients whose immunity is still active respond to the vaccine. Inactivated cancer cells are often combined with BCG to direct the stimulated defense system to recognize tumor cells and fight them, it is claimed.

It seems to me that it is entirely rational to state that the reason the BCG vaccine is effective not only against tuberculosis but leprosy as well as cancer is because of the fact that the Progenitor *Cryptocides* is closely related to the BCG since it is in the same family, the Actinomycetales. This may also explain why, in some cases, Krebiozen (now called Carcalon) is effective in varying degrees since the *Actinomyces bovis* used to stimulate the RES of the horse is also related. The method of extracting the *Actinomyces bovis* for stimulating the immune system could prove to be of inestimable value to man if this method were used to extract BCG or the *Cryptocides*. The efficacy of the killed autogenous vaccines that we use could very well be surpassed either by the use of attenuated strains or by potent extracts, which might stimulate the RES directly if the patient can still respond immunologically. If not, he could receive the passively produced material from serum of animals immunized with the extracts of the *Cryptocides*. It is reported from London that smallpox vaccine has been used in melanoma and in cancer of the cervix. It seems that the inflammation produced by the virus allows cell-killing autoantibodies, macrophages and lymphocytes to get into better contact with the cancer cells, it has been reported in the *British Medical Journal,* May 30, 1970. However, smallpox vaccination is only limited to the site of the vaccination and does not have a systemic effect as does BCG.

Considering the fiasco in which our government participated in the administration of Sabin vaccine which was contaminated with SV-40, a simian tumor agent that produces cancer in experimental animals and probably disease in man, it seems highly ridiculous that the same government is prosecuting physicians, manufacturers and distributors of Laetrile, a nontoxic food supplement. Millions of people were implanted accidentally with SV-40 by vaccines produced under government control. The same neglect occurred in the preparation of the Salk vaccines. Now it is stated that ineffective influenza vaccines have been released through the Division of Biologics Standards. It seems to me that the Federal Drug Administration would do better to attend to more pressing problems within the area of licensure of harmful and dangerous chemicals such as 5 FU and CCNU than to prosecute, if not persecute, the proponents of Laetrile, the generic name for which is nitriloside, cyanophoriglycosides of dietary significance (oil of bitter almonds, which contains the nitrilosides, has been in the U. S. Pharmacopeia for years). One of the most common nitrilosides is amygdalin. The seeds of apples, apricots, cherries, peaches, plums, nectarines and the like carry this factor often in the concentration of 2 to 3 percent. Ernest T. Krebs, Jr. is to be commended on his thoroughness and persistence in studying the chemistry of this material and presenting both to the scientific world and the public the beneficial results of the nitrilosides in producing and maintaining certain important metabolic controls in the human. It is a little known fact that potassium thiocyanate is produced in the normal stomach. Its role in metabolism has never been elucidated. Recently the role of cyanate in the control of sickle-cell anemia has been reported.

The nitrilosides may account for the thiocyanates in the body fluids, as in blood, urine, saliva, sweat and tears, for part of the benzoic acid and subsequently hippuric acid which are saliscylic acid isomers, the material that is aspirin, and also for the hydrocyanic acid that goes to the production of cyanocobalamin from hydrocobalamin or production of vitamin B-12 from provitamin B-12. It would seem that the nitrilosides occurring so abundantly in seeds might also be responsible in some way for regulating the differentiation and maturation of the plant cells as they sprout and differentiate into all their marvelous components. Great oaks from little acorns grow. All of these observations lead to the bone of contention, that the nitrilosides exert some regulatory effect on cancer. As Dr. Dean Burk has so frequently pointed out, the antineoplastic chemotherapeutic agents such as 5 FU and others of the same ilk cause lasting remissions in cancer in only 1.5 per cent while Laetrile is reported to accomplish long-term remissions in 10-15 percent, in addition to alleviating pain and adding months of comfort to the advanced cancer patient.

This harmless material has been banned from interstate commerce in the United States. Even the bitter almonds containing Laetrile (amygdalin) have been removed from the health food stores. How ridiculous can things become? Is the government to dictate to us what harmless substances we may or may not eat? Must the cancer patient be forced to die in pain according to the edicts issued from Washington while suffering the morbidity and destructive effects of the officially and bureaucratically approved chemotherapeutic agents?

It is no wonder that our people flee from this country to Mexico and Europe where they can obtain a number of nontoxic and therapeutic agents not licensed in the United States. They are like leaves driven before the furious hurricane of cancer, seeking relief from pain. One well-known cancer specialist said to me, "I can't understand why they want to go to Mexico.

I always give my patients all the morphine they want." Must the dying patient become a drug addict? All too frequently the terminal patient, his insurance funds and personal assets exhausted, is sent home to die, ignored by the physician who has cut, burned and poisoned him with the admonition, "There is nothing more to do. Call me if you need more medications." At least some foreign physicians offer some alternative to this callous rejection. I liken the boarding homes on the American-Mexican border to waystations or underground shelters for those who are fleeing from the sentence of death. Some of my ancestors gave their lives in helping the slaves escape to freedom in the North and in Canada. Our people are enslaved by ignorance, prejudice, bigotry, and the edicts of a dictatorial and suppressive bureaucratic government. I am not advocating that cancer patients receive Laetrile or endorsing its efficacy in any way. I am endorsing freedom of choice for the informed cancer patient and his inalienable right to choose his medical treatment. It is recommended that all readers get the book *The Dictocrats* by Omar V. Garrison.

There are other competent physicians in Mexico and Canada who have made available many excellent medications licensed in Europe to Americans who have come to them for treatment. These physicians frequently travel extensively every year to the leading clinics of Europe from whence they bring back reports and new methods of treatment with medications licensed in the various European countries. Every effort has been made by the American Cancer Society to harass some of these physicians in the border towns and to drive them out. Fortunately the Mexican government has not always seen fit to follow the American edicts.

Statements From: SIXTH
NATIONAL CANCER CONFERENCE PROCEEDINGS

(Denver Hilton Hotel, Denver Colorado,
September 18–20, 1968, Sponsored by
American Cancer Society, Inc., and
the National Cancer Institute)

J.B. Lippincott Company, July 1970

Although preoperative and postoperative radiation therapy have been used extensively and for decades, it is still not possible to prove an unequivocal clinical benefit from this combined treatment. . . .

Even if the rate of cure does improve with a combination of radiation and therapy, it is necessary to establish the cost in increased morbidity which may occur in patients with or without favorable response to the additional therapy.

> p. 33, William Powers, M.D., Director, Division
> of Radiation and Therapy, Washington
> University School of Medicine, St. Louis,
> Missouri, on "Preoperative and Postoperative
> Radiation Therapy for Cancer."

The thirty year monotonous plateau of the death rate for breast cancer has persisted despite physicians' awareness of breast cancer, refinements of methods of inspecting and palpating the breast, educating women in self-examination, improvements in radiotherapy that include supervoltage, use of more extensive surgical procedures, and the use of chemotherapy and hormones. The enormity of the public-health problem of breast cancer can be realized by considering that: (1) in women the breast is the most common site of cancer, the incidence being higher than that of all malignant neoplasms of the reproductive organs combined; and (2) only approximately one-fourth of the patients with breast cancer survive ten years.

> p. 153, Robert L. Egan, M.D., Professor of
> Radiology, Chief, Mammography Section

Emory University School of Medicine,
Atlanta, Georgia, and R. Waldo Powell, M.D.,
Associate Professor of Surgery, Department
of Surgery, Emory University School of
Medicine, Atlanta, Georgia, on
"Mammography and Diseases of the Breast."

Patients with cancers of the intestine also merit our attention from the viewpoint of prognosis for survival. More than half of those found to have intestinal cancer can be expected to succumb to it in spite of the appearance of numerous therapeutic innovations during the past hundred years. By the time diagnosis is made, the cancer has already spread beyond the confines of the bowel wall and cure is not likely to be achieved for most of these patients.

p. 439, Victor A. Gilbertsen, M.D., University
of Minnesota Medical School,
Minneapolis, Minnesota, on "Bowel
Cancer Detection: Experience with
75,000 Proctosigmoidoscopic
Examinations."

There has been an enormous undertaking of cancer research to develop anticancer drugs for use in the management of neoplastic diseases in man. However, progress has been slow, and no chemical agents capable of inducing a general curative effect on disseminated forms of cancer have yet been developed.

p. 543, Robert D. Sullivan, M.D., Department
of Cancer Research, Lahey Clinic
Foundation, Boston, Massachusetts,
on "Ambulatory Arterial Infusion in the
Treatment of Primary and Secondary
Skin Cancer."

No virus has as yet been found that indubitably actuates tumors in man."—Peyton Rous, in his 1966 Nobel Lecture (Cancer Research, 27, 1919-1924, Nov. 1967).

Case
Histories

As long ago as November 1954 in the French paper, *"Noir et Blanc"* ("Black and White"), Dr. F. W. Lorenz and Doctor Eva Curie, the daughter of Madame Marie Curie, reported the recovery of a little French boy who had a sarcoma using antitoxin made from the cancer organism as identified in France. Dr. F.W. Lorenz's work is quoted as follows: "The remedy is an antitoxin against the microbe of cancer which develops at first as a blood parasite within the red blood cells and which becomes virulent for various reasons, perhaps increased alkalinity of the blood. Originally in the blood cells it is in a resting, spore stage but on activation, it develops all of its virulent forms including the rod, the sign of malignancy." Dr. Lorenz uses the darkfield microscope blood examinations as a method of prognostication as to the presence of the virulent forms of the cancer organism. He is but one example of the large group of well-known physicians in Europe who are using immunization and antitoxic methods to control the cancer infection. The men who attempted this kind of therapy in this country were outlawed and discredited.

The P. *Cryptocides* organisms are ubiquitous and latent in the human race as well as in animals. In doing a survey of one hundred people chosen more or less at random, 40 percent presented blood from which the organism could be cultured readily, 20 percent could be cultured with difficulty, and 40 percent not at all. All cancer patients and all patients with collagen disease had positive cultures in this study.

If one considers that many members of the human race finally succumb in middle or old age to cancer or one of the collagen diseases it is not surprising to find that the P. *Cryptocides* organism is present in apparently normal individuals. Dr. Diller, as previously mentioned, showed that apparently normal mice, from whose blood similar organisms were cultured, were those that later developed cancerous growths. It seems highly probable that predictive diagnosis could be made in humans by the use of blood and urine cultures and by the examination of the blood using darkfield as well as with specific dye methods in the lightfield microscope. One may ask why collagen and degenerative diseases are grouped with neoplasia. The monumental work of Francisco Duran-Reynals may serve to clarify this point. When he infected susceptible hosts with a neoplastic agent one-third died shortly from toxicity, one-third, with partial immunity, developed tumors, and one-third, while surviving a longer period, developed collagen and degenerative disease. So he interpreted neoplasia as a semi-immune response to an infectious agent. The patient does not have to present the full panoply of his disease in order to demonstrate its presence. There can be all manner of modification of disease in terms of virulence and host resistance.

Many patients with neoplastic disease have been treated for many years by numerous therapeutic methods. The evaluation of the efficacy of treatment has been largely clinical based principally on the obliteration of the tumor mass by various means such as surgery, radiation and/or chemotherapy. The tumors have been graded, the degree and extent of metastases noted; the accessibility to surgery, and the sensitivity to radiation, chemotherapeutic agents and antibiotics have led to fairly reliable prognosis as to the course of the disease in any particular group of individuals. Survival curves and percentages may then be calculated with a fair degree of accuracy for the particular type of tumor, the stage at time of discovery, the age and sex of the patient and the type of treatment administered. However, the difficulty lies not in the percentage of the survival rate but in the predictive recognition of which patients will be the long-term survivors. Success is judged by the absence of recurrence of the tumor as determined by the known diagnostic tools available to the present-day physician. Unfortunately, only the actual recurrence of the tumor heralds the failure of the particular method of treatment employed.

In the cases cited below, the earlier patients received only autogenous vaccines and mandelamine, a mild urinary antiseptic. However, with the passage of time we added other substances such as gamma globulin, Pantigen, enzymes, higher vitamin dosages, transfusions and specific antibiotics monitored by urine cultures and darkfield examinations of blood. All of these methods are used to assist the patients to increase their immune competence. We find that now there is no one suffering from collagen disease who cannot be benefited to some extent by this treatment. However, in some cases, therapy, although helpful cannot really extend useful life such as in the case of a woman who came in recently with a tube hanging from her nose. She was breathing through a hole in her trachea. She carried her liquid diet with her in a bottle and a syringe to put it into the tube. She still had hope that she would recover. Her physician had told her that by Valentine's day she would be swallowing again normally. After checking her over carefully, it was obvious that her entire pharynx was filled with cancer. I suspected that her esophagus was largely removed and all she had was a plastic tube going into her stomach. When I called her physician by long distance telephone to ask him for confirmation of these facts, he said very reluctantly that these findings were true but he "Just didn't want to tell her or her husband" what the real situation was. We couldn't refuse to help her, but we felt completely frustrated and inadequate. It was like putting a band-aid on a compound fracture.

On another occasion a heavy, short woman was brought into the office in a wheelchair. She could move her head and her left arm and hand slightly. She was accompanied by her husband and brother. She, her brother and her father all had cancer of the nasopharynx. The father had died. The brother was still going to business but he had multiple metastases in the skeleton. She had received very heavy radiation over the area of the cervical spine and neck, which resulted in her becoming paralyzed. Her physician put her in the hospital and said that if she were fattened up the coverings on her nerves in her neck would regrow and she would recover from her paralysis. All that had happened was that she gained fifty pounds making it much more difficult for her rather small husband to give her complete care.

Still another patient, a marine colonel, came with a huge abdomen due to a swollen liver. He was just a skeleton. His wife begged us to do something, anything. He had been an Eagle Scout, owned a large business, and had been decorated many times in the war. He was a wonderful man only fifty years old. Our nurse said that she thought we should ask them to leave as quickly as possible because she thought he would die in the office. However, we could not refuse him help. We worked very hard with him. His liver went down considerably, he gained some body weight and became much more comfortable. Later, after treatment, he reported that he was able to take his family on a little vacation for a few days. He survived several more months and finally died quietly at home.

We do not like to say who is to be helped and who is not to be but sometimes in spite of the family's urging, a patient will say that there is just not enough left to live for and there is no motivation to try to go on with life. Some of these people could continue for a number of months but they prefer to go to bed, stop eating and take maximum doses of drugs. Others, who are desperately ill and literally ready to die, will cling tenaciously to life and follow every direction minutely. These are the cases that wring the heart with grief. We accepted a terminal patient with cancer of the pancreas, because he was the brother of a friend. It seemed that he would die in a day or two as he was completely jaundiced, had had no bowel movements in ten days, was bloated with swelling of the extremities and face, and hadn't been able to eat for two weeks due to nausea. We had him transfused and started him on nonspecific therapy. That is six weeks ago. He is now eating, his bowels are moving, his jaundice has lightened and he is feeling stronger. However, his pain is still extremely severe. I do not feel that he can have a favorable outcome but we are committed to helping him in any way that we can.

Also by trying to assist the desperately ill we can develop additional experience and information as to the best methods of treatment. Sometimes, a patient who seems completely hopeless will go into a remission. When this happens, all of our efforts are rewarded. The following are actual reports:

1. V.C.—A fifty-six-year-old white woman had a left radical mastectomy September 28, 1965. The pathological diagnosis was mucinous adenocarcinoma of the left breast with invasion into the chest wall. A rib resection was done with a plastic repair at the site of the tumor. Following surgery she was started by her physician on autogenous vaccine cultures from urine. She was given mandelamine. The urine pH was kept at 6 or under. She received treatment regularly until two years ago at which time she took treatment only intermittently. She is completely well with no recurrences. She has been studied at the University Hospital in San Diego with mammograms as well as skeletal and chest X-rays. She has remained free from disease. She follows a good diet with high vitamin dosage and continues with autogenous vaccines in courses.

2. J.C.—In 1968 this fifty-eight-year-old white male came to live with his daughter in La Jolla because of terminal cancer. He reported that he had five major surgeries between 1964 and 1966 and received cobalt in 1966 for cancer of the colon and rectum and had four colostomy openings later repaired. His culture was found by the laboratory to be sensitive to cephalothin, with which he was treated with injections four times daily for one month. A mass the size of a small grapefruit in the lower abdomen was found to diminish by two-thirds. At the same time an autogenous vaccine was ordered and injections were given twice weekly. Previously he complained of severe and intractable abdominal pain. He was on Darvon every three hours with little or no relief. Studies by neurologists were of little help. Roentgen examination revealed a wire mesh used to strengthen the abdominal wall. He said his pain diminished markedly on treatment. He returned when the tumor became operable to New York City where Dr. George Pack of Memorial Hospital removed the now operable tumor and repaired the abdominal wall eliminating the metal wire. He was advised to stop the mandelamine and the autogenous vaccine and dietary restrictions. This advice he followed. His family said he continued active and well and worked another six months, when the tumor recurred and he died a few months later in Texas.

3. R.W.O.—This forty-six-year-old white male was in good health in May 1961 with the exception of permanent skeletal and neurological damage suffered in an automobile accident in 1952. In October 1961 a mass was discovered in his chest about 3 x 4 cm in the mediastinum. He was admitted to the U.S. Naval Hospital in San Diego where additional examinations showed that the tumor was growing rapidly. It was then the size of a tennis ball. On surgery the mass extended around the great vessels of the mediastinum and into the heart muscle. Biopsy only was done since the tumor was inoperable. The pathological diagnosis was malignant thymoma. One course of cobalt was given. A total of 6500 R was completed in March 1962. An

autogenous vaccine was made and he was started on that in December 1961 along with mandelamine, to which his infection was sensitive, and the prescribed diet with high vitamin intake. He said he did well and continued to work until the summer of 1971 when he suffered paroxysmal tachycardia with congestive heart failure. He developed a pleural effusion of about 1000 cc, which was drawn off and carefully studied. There was no evidence of tumor. He restarted active treatment and received vaccine. He continues intermittently on the autogenous vaccine and is on diminishing amounts of medication for his cardiac condition. He says he is doing well and working regularly as a dentist.

4. G.D.—This thirty-seven-year-old white male master mechanic with the USN submarine service was admitted to the U.S. Naval Hospital because of severe headaches December 7, 1964. A month previously he had been in a car accident and was shaken up considerably. December 16, 1964, he was operated on and an infilterating astrocytoma grade II was subtotally resected from the right frontal lobe. He developed a wound abscess with recurrent fluid which refused to heal. VWCL was asked to see the patient. Cultures from the wound consisted of coccal bodies which when cultured proved to be a form of P. *Cryptocides*. He was treated with Keflin and mandelamine at Naval Hospital and the wound healed. He was assigned to light duty at the time and started on autogenous vaccine. He says he did well until a localized mass appeared at the operative site elevating the scalp. He was reoperated on in May 1966. The tumor was well walled off by encapsulation and did not appear to have spread. The right middle cerebral artery was severed accidentally at surgery and he developed a left-sided hemiparesis. He continued on the autogenous vaccine, prescribed diet and vitamins. Except for the paralysis he claimed he did very well for the eighteen months he remained here. The family then left San Diego to live in another state. He was no longer under supervision and discontinued all treatment and died two years later. The interesting

feature of this case was that the tumor which was draining in the beginning, healed and walled off completely as seen on subsequent surgery. Sections of the tumor at the second surgery showed the center of the tumor to be a mass of interlacing mycelial threads and acid-fast bodies with a strong encapsulating fibrous wall.

5. C.M.—In 1965 a white male twenty-one years old was diagnosed to have Hodgkins's disease of the skin, which is extremely rare, and apparently terminates in disseminated reticulum cell sarcoma. He was seen a number of times by the dermatological society, and the biopsy sections were studied by a number of the leading pathologists in the United States. He has been on autogenous vaccines for five years. The course has been variable. On some occasions the diffuse tumors of the anterior chest wall have almost disappeared, only to swell and become red again after some months. At present the tumors appear to have largely subsided. He has also been treated with suitable antibiotics, vitamins and dietary adjuvants.

6. D.G.—This white woman age forty had a total thyroidectomy for cancer in 1964. In August 1970 she was very weak, easily fatigued and was drinking up to thirty cups of coffee daily to keep going. She was also on replacement thyroid. She showed a moderate anemia and a sedimentation rate of 38. Other blood chemistries were within normal limits. Examination of her blood by darkfield and vital stain with the light microscope showed a massive invasion of her red cells with only a few not involved. Many other pleomorphic forms in the blood were present in abundance. She was treated with diet, autogenous vaccine, antibiotics, immune globulines, non-specific white-cell stimulants and rest. She says she felt better. Her sedimentation rate dropped to 14, blood chemistries became normal, strength improved. She secured a job in another state, continues on her vaccine and says she is feeling well.

7. D.K.—A seventy-one-year-old white male operated on for carcinoma of the prostate, followed by an orchidectomy July 7,

1966. He had multiple spinal metastases and arthritis of many joints. He was barely able to move around. He was placed on autogenous vaccine and mandelamine, 1 gram four times a day with dietary and vitamin adjuvants. Previous to his prostatic surgery he had a bowel resection for cancer of the colon. At the present time the spinal metastases have healed, he says he has no evidence of arthritis, is in perfect health and working at his business.

8. T.B.—This forty-two-year-old woman brought her daughter in with terminal Hodgkin's disease in 1968. She did not respond to any treatment and died shortly thereafter. The mother, who had nursed her daughter during this terminal illness, showed a very heavy microbic growth in the urine, indicating a loss of immunity. She was advised to have an autogenous vaccine made which she used prior to the time of her daughter's death. She was carefully observed for signs of neoplasia. Six months after the daughter's death in 1967 she felt two breast masses. Biopsies were taken and the right one about 2 cm in diameter was found to be malignant. She was very depressed and against all medical advice refused to have a mastectomy performed. She has continued on the vaccine ever since. Repeated examinations and mammagrams by Dr. Marshall Milton of San Diego have shown no evidence of recurrence of the breast cancer to date.

9. S.G.—This New York woman has had many cancer incidents in her life. Radical breast surgery 1932, a hysterectomy for cancer of the uterus in 1940, and in May 1965 surgery for cancer of the other breast. All during the years she has taken a variety of nonspecific vaccines and antibiotics. In 1965 an autogenous vaccine was made to which she reacted somewhat violently, but continued on the therapy after it was diluted. At present she is in excellent health and presents only a scant growth of the organism in the blood and urine showing a rise in her immune response.

10. S.W.—This white female from Nevada, age forty-one, had a left radical mastectomy in 1961. In the interval she had a child. In 1965 she had widespread bone metastases and an oophorectomy was performed. She was started on male hormones which did not agree with her and were promptly discontinued. We first saw her in 1966 at which time she received autogenous vaccines, cephalin, vitamins and diet. Following two months of therapy she had a good regression of the lesions with filling in of the femoral heads and some of the lesions of the spine and skull. A report from Dr. David A. Adams, radiologist, dated June 5, 1967, states, "there has been definite filling in of the lesions in the frontal region of the skull since the previous examination. The osteolytic areas are smaller and new bone formation has bridged between them."

At the time she presented herself, she stated that she was advised to have a bilateral adrenalectomy which she refused. She remained on autogenous vaccines and adjuvants very comfortably for five years. She lived in an isolated area out of this state and it was difficult to keep in close touch with her. At the end of five years she began to deteriorate. At this time she had the adrenalectomy performed and died within the month.

11. R.A.G.—White female forty-six years old was suffering, in 1965, with generalized carcinomatosis when referred to us. March 1962 she had a right radical mastectomy followed by cobalt. Her mother died in 1963 of leukemia. They lived together. In 1964 showers of fibromata appeared over the trunk. December 8, 1964, a left mastectomy was done, with cancer cells found throughout all the breast tissue. Bilateral oophorectomy was performed December 22, 1964. The peritoneum was peppered with nodules. She was on thiotepa and testosterone for three months. Mandelamine was started February 2, 1965, and March 1965, she was started on autogenous vaccine. She said she improved remarkably and took an eight-week trip to Scandinavia. On return she was able to care for her home and work at her business. In 1966, she developed herpes

ophthalmicus and received heavy steroid treatment. Her blood picture worsened at this time but by July 1966 she was working full time after continuing vaccine and adjuvants. January 1967, the bone survey was negative and she said she continued to do well. Late in 1969 she developed ascites, had a number of chemical intrapertoneal injections without improvement and she died six months later.

12. G.S.—He is a sixty-eight-year-old white male operated on May 5, 1971. He had adenocarcinoma right parotid gland with poorly differentiated metastatic nodes at all levels of the right side of the neck and upper thorax. Laboratory examination June 4, 1971, showed a secondary anemia and high glucose with a low total protein and albumen. These were all corrected at the next examination in six weeks. Cultures were taken for autogenous vaccine May 15, 1971. He was followed with darkfield and vital staining examinations of his blood and periodic urine cultures. Treatment was given according to the results of these examinations. He received as medication: autogenous vaccine, placental gamma globulin, pantigen sorbitrate, streptomycin, tetracycline, lincomycin, mandelamine, gantrisin and avazyme, Synthroid, bacid, erythromycin, myambutal, vitamins, $Mg.Cl_2$ 10% and analgesics as indicated. He improved sufficiently to go back East to the Atlantic coast for two weeks at the end of October 1971. He says he is doing well and working at the present time. His physician says he has no recurrence and urine cultures are negative. Dark field examinations of the blood show no virulent forms but the latent bodies are still present in small numbers. At a recent checkup by his referring physician he was told that he is in excellent health.

Cases by cooperating physicians:

1. C.C.—This fifteen-year-old white female high school student was first operated on June 23, 1964. A right oophorectomy was performed. The pathological diagnosis was "malignant cystic

teratoma." She did not do well and was reoperated on January 18, 1965, at which time she had widespread abdominal metastases. A mass the size of a grapefruit was removed. On February 1, 1965, cobalt 60 was started but the patient stopped after two treatments. She was started on autogenous vaccine by her physician and continued until August 24, 1967, and intermittently since then. Recent examination shows no evidence of tumor. She has now completed college, teaches school and says she is in excellent health. She continues with her diet. Her urine cultures are negative.

2. M.F.—She had a right radical mastectomy, March 3, 1965. Pathological diagnosis, "undifferentiated carcinoma." Autogenous vaccine was made and treatment was given from May 9, 1965 through November 9, 1966, and intermittently since. Her physician states that urine cultures and physical checkups through 1971 show no evidence of recurrence.

3. J.M.—White female age thirty-five had a left radical mastectomy March 3, 1965, when four months pregnant. Pathological diagnosis was infiltrating carcinoma, scirrhus and medullary types. After delivery of a normal child at term she had a hysterectomy May 28, 1965, and was placed on estrogen therapy from August 24, 1966, through January 9, 1967. Autogenous vaccine was made which she took for a year and intermittently since. This type of tumor is universally fatal. Her physician says she is in good health at the present time (1972) with no signs of recurrence.

4. O.B.—White female age fifty had a radical mastectomy May 16, 1963. Pathological diagnosis was medullary carcinoma. She had radiation to breast and ovaries. Her physician gave her autogenous vaccine September 1, 1965, to July 27, 1967, and intermittently since. Present condition excellent, according to her physician.

5. K.B.—White female age fifty-four had a right mastectomy September 29, 1965. Pathological diagnosis was carcinoma of

the right breast, ductal type, with metastatic carcinoma to two of six axillary lymph nodes. Autogenous vaccine was given November 19, 1965, through August 15, 1967, and intermittently since then. Last urine cultures were negative. July 29, 1967, hospitalized for bowel obstruction—not malignant. She was operated, recovered, and is now working full time in 1972, according to her physician.

6. F.B.—White male age twenty-seven from Utah, who was operated for severe headaches after a number of convulsive seizures. The pathological diagnosis was astrocytoma, grade III to IV, infiltrating the surrounding area. He received anticonvulsants, radiotherapy and antibiotics. In 1966 when he was doing very badly and appeared to be terminal, he was placed on autogenous vaccines and mandelamine, one gram four times daily, plus vitamins and dietary supplements. He remained on this regimen for two years. The vaccine was discontinued in October 1970. His physician said there is no evidence of any tumor at present. However, he is maintained on anticonvulsants.

7. K.H.—White male nineteen years of age was operated 1965 for a complete obstruction C5 through T2 of the spine. Pathological diagnosis was cystic astrocytoma of the spinal cord. He was started on autogenous vaccine in 1966 and has remained on it ever since. He has done very well, his physician says, and maintained the same status he had on discharge from the hospital. The preoperative paralysis is unchanged except for the use of his arms, which has improved, and he can now walk with some assistance. There is no evidence of recurrence of the tumor, it is said.

8. D.K.—A forty-six-year-old longshoreman of Oriental extraction was operated on July 20, 1967, for a mass on the right side of his neck. Pathological diagnosis was malignant lymphoma, reticulum-cell type with invasion of all glands. These were not resectable because they extended under the sternocleidomastoid muscle and into the chest cavity. He received a course of X-ray,

4500 R, in eighteen treatments. Since then he has had no other treatment except autogenous vaccine continuously with erythromycin 250 mgm twice a day. The microorganisms remain sensitive to erythromycin. He says he is completely well and works full time on the docks. His blood picture still shows some parasitization but in a state of latency.

9. R.A.—A mature adult white male had carcinoma of the prostate with extension into the bladder. After surgery he was put on autogenous vaccine in 1965 which he has continued since. He had a slight fibrous recurrence of the tumor in the bladder which was successfully resected. He also had metastases to the spine which are now completely healed. He was on standard female hormone therapy for a few years but has discontinued this therapy and is taking only the autogenous vaccine. As of 1971 he is said to be free of tumor or evidence of metastasis.

10. E.W.—White female sixty-six years old was operated for a breast tumor 1965. Pathological diagnosis, necrotic anaplastic medullary-type duct-cell carcinoma with no evidence of extension to any of the lymph nodes. She was started on the autogenous vaccine in 1965 after surgery and has continued with it ever since. She continues in excellent health with no evidence of recurrence.

Recent cases treated with combined therapy:

Sometimes we are obliged to treat patients who are receiving many other forms of therapy. Here is a report of five of these cases:

1. K.Y.—In ten years this man had seven operative procedures to his scalp for epithelioma and squamous cell carcinoma. Each time the tumor was removed more tissue was excised and a larger skin graft was necessary. We were talked into accepting him as a patient by our friend, Mrs. Betty O. He had a four-inch cancer on his head surrounded by nodules which apparently had

grown into his skull. He smoked and he drank. He had developed a devil-may-care attitude for which we didn't blame him. We had to convince him that he needed to change his ways. On treatment the ugly mass cleaned up around the edges, the skin improved and after several months the tissues healed sufficiently so that he became operable. After an eight-hour surgery in which he received a synthetic piece of skull about six inches across he was skin grafted and received a few kernels of radioisotope gold over one area of the brain. He is now healed and well and back to operating an art school. He invited us all to a "Love-In" recently. His doctors, nurses and friends who had generously given blood were all at the party. He was our star. Except for a saber-like scar across the top of his head and some deep scars on his neck, he looked fine and was playing tennis again. He facetiously claimed he had been a Heidelberg graduate and had received his scars while dueling for a lady's honor. He complained that one eyelid drooped a little and he couldn't wiggle one ear too vigorously. His cultures are negative. We do not anticipate any recurrence.

2. J.E.—Again we were prevailed upon to accept a young wife and mother with acute myelogenous leukemia. She had been in the UCLA Medical Center for one month and discharged with the prognosis of one month to live. The Billy Casper family asked us to try to help her. Her hematologist was reluctant to cooperate with us. However, we gave her full immune therapy. In addition, she received brief courses of one 100 mg Purinthal tablet daily and 20 mg. methotrexate intramuscularly weekly. The last three bone-marrow examinations are entirely normal. She was told that there is no evidence of her disease at this time. It is now nearly a year. She says she is completely well, never tired, takes complete care of two young children and her husband. Her hematologist said now that she is so well, he would like to increase the chemicals. We have argued bitterly. I say she doesn't need them and more might be harmful. He says

now that she has done well, maybe she can take a great deal more. We compromised by giving her minimal doses in courses.

3. R.S.—This twenty-five-year-old man came to us with terminal Hodgkin's disease. Practically all of his lymph nodes were involved. He had his spleen removed, received all the chemicals he could tolerate with a full course of radiation. He was vomiting constantly and was brought to our office lying down on a mattress in a station wagon. We followed our usual course of treatment except that he did not receive transfusions. Since he was vomiting we gave him extremely large doses of bicillin intramuscularly because his organisms were sensitive to penicillin. He received all the other recommended therapy. He said within hours the pain in the glands began to subside. We started treating him on January 27, 1972. Today his glands have subsided 90 percent, he has gained eighteen pounds and has gone back to work full time. We hope that he can continue the bicillin without his organisms developing resistance or his acquiring an allergic reaction to the penicillin. We were advised to continue the bicillin for six months. He is working regularly now full time, he says, without any disability. His glands are still somewhat swollen.

4. This forty-year-old wife and mother came to us because she was completely inoperable. She had a large mass in the abdomen from an ovarian carcinoma which had metastasized to the intestines. Even a colostomy was not feasible since the disease was diffuse as found on surgery. She also had one breast completely filled with cancer with metastatic nodes not only in the neck on the involved side but on the opposite side as well. The members of her church fasted and prayed forty-eight hours. She was administered to by the Elders. She had even gone to Tijuana and obtained some Laetrile which she was taking. She was placed on immune therapy as well. In just two weeks the breast tumor had diminished 75 percent and the hardness in her abdomen had subsided. She has normal bowel movements again. The improvement continues to the present time, she says. Her

blood picture is still poor and she is still growing some bacterial colonies from urine but she says that she is feeling better. I would hesitate to say where the credit belongs. Perhaps the medications are not needed where prayer is sufficient. However, we know we must help ourselves as best we can. She still has some residual abdominal pain and is being followed carefully by her referring physician.

5. This young lady of thirty-two had removal of her breast only because at the time of discovery of her breast cancer she had liver and spleen involvement. She had many nodules popping up every few days in her mediastinum or in her neck or under her arm. These nodes were being chased around by the cobalt machine. One would disappear but two more would come. On immune therapy, mild chemicals and radiation, all lesions have gone and the liver has diminished 50 percent in size. She was not getting a favorable response, she says, until she received immune treatment. It is questionable what her final outcome will be.

In accordance with the opinion of numerous medical authorities and after reading all the pertinent literature available a variety of supportive and immune promoting measures have been proposed for these patients. The method for producing the vaccines from body fluids and tissues has been given. The elimination of focal infections and the use of vaccines for these infections have also been described. In addition, adjuvants such as a prescribed diet, high in vitamin content, replacement enzymes, leukocyte stimulators, gamma globulin and combinations of indicated antibiotics were used. Methods of determining the course of the chronic underlying infection by serial cultures as well as by lightfield and darkfield examinations of fresh blood are demonstrated. A selected number of case histories has been related.

The described method of therapy is proposed for the treatment of immune incompetence occurring in neoplastic disease because it is physiologic and based upon immunological procedures. In all cases, especially the terminals, the benefit may not be of great duration but pain can be alleviated and a sense of well-being restored to some degree. In a few cases, especially in young people, the disease appears to regress. In others, the underlying chronic disease may be suppressed, adding months and even years of usefulness to life. In still others, the remission appears permanent although the blood picture indicates a state of latency.

These studies are presented in an effort to indicate and suggest what might be accomplished in the future with the hope that other physicians and research scientists will continue these pertinent investigations toward a common goal. Such a combined effort may well result in the treatment of neoplasia by immunization techniques, preferably preventive, and by utilizing passive immune bodies such as specific antisera and antitoxins when the disease is present. More efficient methods may be developed for employing known antibiotics in larger doses or in combinations that may be more suppressive of the disease. There should be a continued search for new antibiotics as well as reevaluation of old ones that have been shelved.

Cancer
and Politics

More than two billion dollars have been spent for cancer research in the past twenty years. Plans are now under way to spend one billion dollars a year until the conquest of cancer is complete. The target date is July 4, 1976. Congressman John Rooney suggested the control and cure of cancer by 1976 as "an appropriate commemoration of the two hundredth anniversary of the independence of our country." Wonderful if it can be done. Biological problems are hardly solved by political enthusiasm. We do, however, have the example of the atomic bomb and its effect on almost every phase of our lives achieved by a great crash program with unlimited money available to well-prepared scientists with a determination to succeed. The space program is another example. With billions of dollars and an army of skilled and dedicated men the end was achieved. It is asserted that since we can put a man on the moon we can conquer cancer on earth. With these arguments the crash program can be voted and funded. But conquering cancer may be even a more difficult task and there are those who have their doubts about doing it in this way.

Cancer has afflicted mankind since his existence upon the earth. From past experience, the very diagnosis of cancer is a sentence of death, slow and painful to the end. It strikes in the dark, attacks any part of the body and invades and destroys any and all of the organs and tissues, imperceptibly advancing until its victims are doomed even before they are aware that they have this dread and fatal disease. No one is immune to its attack, both sexes and all ages, all classes of society and all races of mankind fall before its onslaught. If we have a dozen people in a room, three will die of cancer and four will suffer with it. Every individual will be challenged by this killer either personally or in his own family or among his close friends. It has a great political impact, and shrewd politicians take advantage of any opportunity it presents. How does this affect the patient? Unless the victim has good insurance coverage or is very wealthy this disease comes as a catastrophe in more ways than one. Financially it is ruinous. One of our patients with acute myelogenous leukemia paid $8,000 for one month of treatment in the hospital at UCLA Medical Center. Another patient after six unsuccessful surgeries spent more than $12,000 in three months and was in the hospital less than three weeks. In the Scandinavian countries and others where medicine is completely socialized the victims of this disease have to do exactly as they are told or further treatment is refused them. The same is probably true in this country for those on welfare and for those who have spent their life's savings and are destitute because of the expense of this disease. The wealthy have a choice of skilled physicians both home and abroad and a choice of the type of treatment. Some go to Europe for specific vaccines and cell therapy and visit the spas where special diets, medications and therapies are available. They have choices. This does not mean that they are always more effectively treated. Money may not buy a cure, but it at least provides a choice of treatment.

And what of the American Cancer Society? What does it do for the patient with the millions of dollars that it collects annually? One of my good friends who headed the American Cancer Society drive in his city remarked wryly, "We send them x thousands of dollars and they send us back a couple hundred pounds of printed matter."

In our system of government, the president may suggest, and then Congress makes the appropriations. This is where lobbies and influence go to work. Note the skill and success of Mary Lasker and her group. Most of the appropriations are granted to the NIH and its ten subdivisions. The funds are used to operate hospitals and for research facilities. Grants are also made to cooperative research groups around the country.

There is lots of competition, infighting and jockeying for positions of power, influence and money where so much of each is available for those shrewd and strong enough to take them. Three years ago we went to a college reunion for one of the well-known colleges, which appears to turn out large numbers of successful graduates. Many of the alumni came in their well-appointed yachts from New York and New England headed for the Florida waters to spend the winter. They stopped off en route for the class reunion. As the social hour got under way and the liquid refreshments flowed freely the talk became free and easy. These successful career men, some with government positions, told of their struggles to get to the top and how they spent more time working for advancement than they ever did on the jobs to which they were assigned.

The Bureau of Narcotics and Dangerous Drugs (BNDD) is a good example of hierarchical bureaucracy. In the *Medical Tribune*, February 23, 1972, is an article entitled "101 Top Scientists Charge U.S. Government Erects 'Barriers to Research' by Its Politics." In a telegram to President Nixon three Nobel laureates and ninety-eight scientists charged the Justice Department with erecting barriers to research and even bringing research to a halt in the name of fighting drug abuse. Rules and regulations with multitudinous forms are drawn up in quadruplicate, numbered perhaps for a computer but so confusing that even a career man from his own department would have difficulty in ordering the most simple of supplies. The new bureau (BNDD) is usurping the authority from the Department of Health, Education and Welfare, which formerly functioned to aid research rather than frustrate and confuse it with the new complex and intricate regulations. When the scientist gets through the paper work he will have neither time nor energy to get anything done with the research. "If you want a gram of marijuana, you have to keep it in a 750-pound safe. If the safe weighs less than that it has to be rooted in cement. Justice Department agents have been making site visits to every researcher in the country to inspect the safes." A gram is about one-fourth of a teaspoonful. To add to the paper work a research protocol, at least in duplicate, has to accompany the application for Schedule 1 substances (dangerous narcotics). If more items are needed the paper work is repeated for each one. Neil L. Chayet, a Boston attorney, and lecturer in legal medicine at Boston University Law School and Tufts Medical School says, "The forms are so complex and there are so many numbers that I do not see how anyone without specialized legal training can interpret them and fill them out properly." My nurse, a supervisor, quit her job at one of the well-known local rest homes because she was so busy counting pills three times a day for the BNDD that she didn't have time to take care of the patients.

A number of leading scientists and teachers in the United States show a growing concern for the therapeutic gap resulting from the American drug regulatory policies of the Food and Drug Administration which they suggest needs a complete overhaul (*Medical Tribune & Medical News*—April 5, 12, 1972). Dr. Robert Dripps, Vice President of Medical Affairs, University of Pennsylvania, says "In England a third of the new drugs now in use have been introduced in the last five years. In this country the corresponding figure is about 10 percent. In the four-year period from 1966 to mid-1971 there were seventy products on the market in England not available to practicing physicians here. Many of these are not important therapeutic agents, but if there is only one vital agent available in England and not available here, it is one too many. Japan and Italy are also making great progress in drug research."

This group of scientists besides Dr. Dripps, includes Dr. Michael E. De Bohey, President of Baylor College of Medicine, Dr. Dickinson W. Richards, Nobelist and Professor of Medicine, Emeritus, Columbia University, and Alfred Gilman, Ph.D., Chairman, Department of Pharmacology, Albert Einstein College of Medicine. They also point out that American medicine now faces a "paradox" in which the drug industry's research capacity is getting better, the FDA is working harder, but there is decreased productivity.

A notation may be made about the "drug inserts," short descriptions of the drugs, their uses, contradictions and complications, ordered by the FDA to accompany each package of drugs. How significant are they and what is the legal status? Do they replace the U.S. Pharmacopeia? What is the responsibility of the drug producer and the physician? About four years ago in the *Archives of Internal Medicine* (AMA publication) a two-page article appeared giving a very comprehensive discussion of one particular drug, listing all complications. On reading it one doctor remarked, "You would have to be crazy to prescribe this." The drug was aspirin. This points up a difficult problem of judgment for the FDA, the manufacturer, the physician and the patient. A recent survey showed that half of the older patients do not take their medicine at all. On the other hand there are those who say, "if a little is good more is better" and they double or triple the dose. Then there were some of the clinic patients receiving treatment at Bellevue Hospital in New York who would take their week's supply as soon as they got out of the clinic, throw the bottle in the gutter and then come back the next week for more medicine.

FDA Commissioner Dr. Charles Edwards describes some of their problems (*Medical Tribune*, April 5, 1972) "We are on the one hand criticized for being 'soft' on industry and, on the other hand called repressive, an enemy of free enterprise; on every major disease we are accused by some of acting too fast without sufficient evidence and by others of acting too slowly and too timidly to prevent unnecessary harm."

The scientists conclude: "We believe a change in the drug regulatory system is badly needed. The system too often stifles creativity and escalates the cost of research; perpetuates a continuing decline in the number of new drugs entering the market in this country and may be depriving the practicing physician of agents beneficial to patient care. The reasons for all this are not clear, are undoubtedly complex, and require thorough investigation and study."

In *Medical Opinion*, January 1972, Dr. Charles L. Mengis discusses public relations, showmanship and selling of various types of expensive, sophisticated periodic examinations. He emphasizes two points: 1) These productions are expensive, requiring institutional or government financing, performed in institutions or hospitals, where they gain an aura of respectability that they do not merit; 2) They often arouse the enthusiasm of laymen who have no insight into their value and judge them by impressiveness and the amount of money and publicity they bring the institution. "We flounder in an ever-widening sea of words and machines, most of which will seem superfluous to the physicians of tomorrow." There is a tremendous drive toward large well-funded centers with good public relations and publicity departments implying that only in these institutions can adequate services be obtained. In reality the patients would do better for their overall health care in local medical centers. Sometimes the famous centers are built around the reputation of one man, who is so busy with public relations work that the patients never get to see him. We are "caught between the push and pull of well-funded lobbyists, ego maniacs, grant-eaters, and mistaken legislators. We small indi viduals may well succumb to collectivization, herded into groups for standardization of therapy, pay and thought."

The following aphorisms are applicable to this program: "Most books are written by writers; most work is done by doers, and they don't talk to each other." "Research is strongly encouraged but only within the framework of the accepted ideology."—American Cancer Association.

Dr. Robert J. Huebner, one of the world's leading virologists, Director of the Viral Disease Laboratory at the National Institute of Health, with headquarters at the Cancer Institute, is in charge of the budget that supports 90 percent of the virology work scattered around the country. This puts him in the bureaucratic and scientific center of cancer research. In 1968 he said, "The basic breakthroughs have already been made." Understanding the cell and how it works is so "exciting that the scientists can't sleep at night just thinking about it." He is a career man and most of his life has been spent with NIH in the field of virology. His clinical experience is perhaps mostly with his prized Aberdeen Angus cattle. He is a controversial man and a branch chief at NCI. "He has the PR instinct of a politician, the fervor of a Billy Graham, and he travels constantly publicizing his ideas" (*Saturday Evening Post,* August 24, 1968). He is one of the best known and strongest backers of the Crash Program.

Dr. Huebner's theory on cancer consists of a theoretical C-particle (probably DNA) which he calls an oncogene. This passes from generation to generation in the genetic material. Originally it was RNA but in some way got into the DNA template, where it is inactive or "switched off" and is a passenger in the genetic material from generation to generation. Then he claims that it is "switched on" by some of the carcinogens, by chemical agents, cigarettes, infection, trauma or some other unknown factors, when it may actively alter the genetic pattern of the cells and produce the malignant changes we call cancer. The oncogene supposedly comes from a virus but after twenty years of research and expenditures of many million of dollars no such "virus" has ever been found connected with human cancer. However, L-forms, mycoplasma and filter-passing tumor agents have all been causally related to cancer formation. These have been observed in the electron microscope and have been successfully used for producing immunization in susceptible animal hosts. If the causative agent is a permanent and inseparable constituent of the cell, then it is hard to explain how immunization can work.

The theories of Nello Mori, of Naples, quoted from *Der Krebsarzt*, Volume 4, pages 309-313 (1949), states that "In view of the modern ideas of the endogenetic cause of cancer I should like to mention that since the beginning of bacteriological investigation Rappin (since 1887) claimed the endocellular genesis and corroborated it with his own investigations. According to Portier, the mitochondria, which he believes to be symbiontic microorganisms, cannot any longer exercise their regulating function due to disturbance of the intracellular balance and this is the cause of the disorganized cell growth.

"I have been thinking for a long time that the tumors are caused by physiological cell symbionts. These microbes attain parasitic properties caused by some external or internal disturbances of the balance between them and the host cell. One would be able to explain easily many heretofore unknown details of tumor genesis with this 'Symbio-parasitic' hypothesis. Most of all one has to stress the fact that a physiological symbiosis of polymorphous mycetes, especially blastomycetes and the body cells of invertebrates, is very well known, which occurs in the cell in ultramicroscopic form. Wallin was able to isolate mitochondria from the lungs of newborn rabbits. Furthermore, Pierantoni, the discoverer of the hereditary endosymbiosis, identified the deuteroplasmatic corpuscles in the yolk of viridis [sic] as microorganisms that can be cultured. After the yolk is used up there is a transition into the ultramicroscopic latent stage. This phase occurs in mature cells. With the development of the new embryo the whole cycle starts all over again.

"When the transition of the microorganisms from the physiological endosymbiontic stage to the parasitic stage takes place, this will cause the formation of antibodies, but not to the extent produced by a bacterium, which enters the body as an alien element. This would explain why it is so difficult to find specific antibodies to the microorganisms that we presume to be the causative agent of carcinoma. Rondoni feels that the carcinoma antibodies are being hidden by a very wide zone of unspecific reactions. It is very difficult, too, to prove the existence of specific antibodies in mycoses and virus diseases."

Does this sound a familiar note? Is Dr. Huebner whistling the tune that Nello Mori wrote?

Another example of research receiving large grants is the work of Renato Dulbecco of the Salk Institute of La Jolla who uses the polyoma virus to study the mechanisms of cell division. His theory depends, in part at least, upon a process called lysogeny, in which a virus called a phage, attacks and infects a bacterium, grows inside the cell and finally kills it. The phage then is free to attack other bacteria. Sometimes the phage attacks the bacteria, and disappears for many generations only to reappear later to reproduce and destroy the bacteria. Dulbecco suggests that the DNA polyoma virus attaches to the DNA of the host cell, and with each cell division there is a replication of both the cell DNA and the polyoma DNA. Cells carrying the polyoma DNA are either cancer cells or potentially cancer cells. This is set up as a prototype. There is, as yet, no viral agent equivalent to the phage, that has been proven to be causative in cancer.

What is needed is a comprehensive study of all known research involving the etiology of cancer and the various modalities of treatment practiced around the world so that the best of this scientific information can be made available to the American public. Basic research, of course, is indispensable but current yet obscure information can be ferreted out, evaluated and if found useful, put into practice. It is futile to retrace the steps of previous investigators and to appropriate their findings in the effort to promote self-interest or self-aggrandizement. We must move forward by utilizing available helpful information, wherever it has originated regardless of the source or the importance of the proponents.

Dr. Irvine H. Page, M.D., in an editorial (*Modern Medicine*, April 19, 1971), "The grand strategy of cancer research," after discussing some of the political aspects has this to say: "The scientist is easily portrayed as an unworldly soul who does not know what is best to do. He needs direction and to be pushed into doing what society really needs by some blue-ribbon authority, commission, or committee appointed by the president himself. That seems almost to guarantee success and make any criticism seem ungrateful and in bad taste." He then points out how great discoveries are made, not by institutions but by individuals, and that the fabulously successful results produced by individual ingenuity are made at an incredibly low price compared with other social endeavors. "The long-range economics of such discoveries as penicillin are incalculable. And oddly, Fleming had neither committee nor large government grants to make it."

Crash programs are no guarantee of good results and frequently the very ideas behind these programs make for ill-conceived research in the "wrong" direction, or with a "hit or miss" shotgun method with the idea that given enough money and enough researchers something good will result. I suggest that the chief result of large appropriations will be an application for more grants and more money to continue the researching indefinitely. The pressure created by inevitably broad publicity of endeavors such as the conquest of cancer encourages scientific opportunism, superficiality and undue competitiveness. The investigator, instead of following his best scientific instinct, is constantly under pressure for a "breakthrough," especially if it can be announced through the mass media shortly before a grant request. Basic research is so expensive that it can only be carried on with grants or gifts, and hopefully without too much waste. Some have suggested that of the billion-dollar grants less than 1 percent will finally be used for honest, sincere, sophisticated, competent, effective research.

Those who administer the grants wield tremendous power and write the rules for the game of "grantsmanship." The successful grantees are usually conservative, avoid "trouble" and listen to the voices of the masters. They first secure their own positions and then become judges of the applicant scientists who propose the prospective research. They can give support to the work or stop it. They can endanger the proponents' standing in the scientific field and ruin the character of those who are so unfortunate as to gain their ill will. Through money they have power. "All power tends to corrupt, and absolute power corrupts absolutely." It is hoped that there will be those who are capable and honest with knowledge in the fields in which they work to do a good job in placing the grants. No one can guarantee that anything good will come out of any particular research project, but the likelihood of success must be weighed. Some people are skeptical of political solutions.

An editorial in the *Medical Tribune*, March 1, 1972, concerning the DeLaney Amendment on carcinogens states: "If microscopic tumors are adjudged malignant then saccharine along with cyclamates would be outlawed. We are not suggesting that saccharine be banned. We question the wisdom of banning cyclamates and suggest that when medical questions are handled as political questions, they are likely to be mishandled."

There are other sources of grants and research money besides the government. A number of foundations contribute to this work, as well as organizations such as the American Cancer Society. Also millions of dollars are contributed annually by private individuals such as Armand Hammer, grantor to the Salk Institute who supports work in which he has a knowledge of the researchers involved and believes the work to be worthwhile. Other work is carried on by dedicated people who work independently giving of their own time, money and effort. In proportion these have been far more productive in many cases then the more generously endowed institutions. However, there are some projects that can only be carried out with the services of a large and well-equipped establishment.

Some rules for getting grants, or grantsmanship

Many scientists apply for grants in established fields. They feel much more secure going along with popular and current ideas. They will have fewer problems and less criticism staying with the thinking of the Establishment.

Helpful rules to obtain grants:

1. Use this year's language. It seems ridiculous that grants would be given or rejected based upon the "terms" that are used. It must sound sophisticated. Some of the effective words are iatrogenic, entropy, parameter, esoteric, serendipity, elegant.

2. Ask for enough money. Some grants have been turned down because the applicants failed to ask for substantial amounts of money. The grantors apparently estimate the importance of the work by the amount of money for which the application is made. Some research may not accomplish much anyway, and the request for a small amount makes them very nervous.

3. Avoid definitive and controversial subjects. Keep the objective in the nebulous, in the gray areas, and avoid the sharply defined activities spelled out in black and white. This gives a wider range of research and failure of accomplishment is not so glaring if what one is doing isn't very clear in the first place.

4. Research is to be strongly encouraged—but only in the framework of the accepted ideology.

Let us hope that political manipulation will eventually result in better care for the cancer patient and the ultimate solution of the cancer problem.

On December 23, 1971, the National Cancer Act of 1971 was signed by President Nixon, titular head of the program. The aims, demonstration and administration all appear noteworthy and could be most effective. Let us hope that it can be potentiated by men of good will and high moral conscience. Let us pray that a period of enlightenment will follow, and the well-known abuses of the FDA will be eliminated so that all available knowledge concerning cancer will be made accessible to the people. May each individual suffering with this dread disease be considered a very special charge, a subject of great concern and not be counted as a unit in the compilation of figures in the attempt to prove the efficacy of toxic and dangerous drugs.

It should be a rule following the recommendation of the Code of Nuremberg that each patient "should have made known to him the nature, duration and purpose of the experiment; method and means by which it is to be conducted; all inconveniences and hazards to be expected; and effect upon his health or person which may possibly come from his participation in the experiment." There is irrefutable evidence that time and time again, experiments carried out by researchers acting under NCI supervision have violated this rule. There is another rule in the Nuremberg Code stating that no experiment shall be conducted where death or disabling disease is expected unless the doctor himself is willing to serve as a subject. The proponent of any new therapy whether for cancer or any other disease should be obliged to show proof that he has taken the medication in a full therapeutic dose for the period of time recommended.

How the new Cancer Act will be administered and its defects

The Code of Nuremberg was set up at the Nuremberg trials at which time four Nazi doctors were tried and hanged with an

American acting as chief prosecutor. The Nuremberg Code was established to protect helpless prisoners of war from harmful medical or surgical experimentation. It states clearly that no experiment shall be conducted where death or disabling disease is expected unless the doctor himself serves as a subject.

Only recently a well-known woman lawyer was found to have widespread cancer of the lung which was inoperable. She was eligible for treatment at Naval Hospital in San Diego, California. She came to consult with us after treatment had been started. She had been given a new, experimental, highly toxic drug called CCNU which, after administration, continues to act for six weeks. It is highly destructive of bone marrow. She had received one dose only of 220 milligrams about the size of half an aspirin tablet. The toxic effects of this small dose was not expected to wear off for six weeks. No one who had received this medication had lived more than fourteen months with lung cancer. Its efficacy is not demonstrable. It is known to be highly toxic. After three weeks it was thought that she could stand another half dose of the drug. Immediately she became violently ill. She came to our office in a dying condition. We could only recommend hospitalization. She was admitted to Naval Hospital where she promptly died. The use of experimental drugs at the government hospitals is under the direct supervision of the Surgeon General of the United States. There is no record to show that he took CCNU himself as is required by the Nuremburg Code for the administration of known toxic drugs.

It is hoped that those individuals charged with the use of these vast amounts of money provided by the taxpayers will forget the past commitments and prejudices of the FDA, the Cancer Society and the AMA. Dr. Hans Morgenthau of the University of Chicago said that the nation may be faced by "rule by a mediocre scientific clique that persists in error to the point of catastrophe." He goes on further to state that scientists and administrators who have made great errors involving large human and material resources are afraid to admit that they are wrong and all these resources are wasted. Major effort may follow major effort until catastrophe takes the place of timely retreat. In thirteen years the NCI has spent five hundred million dollars and has tested 170,000 poisonous drugs for possible use in the fight against cancer. The results have been zero except in a few rare types of cancer. Over 100,000 cancer patients have been used as guinea pigs often without their full knowledge and informed consent.

Let us hope that the FDA will have more pressing and productive business than to bring suit and condemnation against the advocates of harmless nontoxic treatments for cancer and that they will cease to suppress the freedom of the press. On May 3, 1971, Louis F. Saylor, M.D., Director of Public Health of the State of California, as Plaintiff tried to obtain an injunction against the International Association of Cancer Victims and Friends and their officers, editor and publisher as well as against the National Health Federation. The prosecutors attempted to stop publication of their magazines and press releases. This word "press" has been construed down through our history in this country as applying to every means of communication, including verbal, films, writings, pamphlets, books and whatever. It follows that authority is to be controlled by public opinion, not public opinion by authority.

We set up government by consent of the governed, and the Bill of Rights denies those in power any legal opportunity to coerce that consent. The vitality of civil and political institutions in our society depends on free discussion. As Chief Justice Hughes wrote in *De Jonge* vs. *Oregon*: "It is only through free debate and free exchange of ideas that government remains responsive to the will of the people and peaceful change is effected. The right to speak freely and to promote diversity of ideas and programs is therefore one of the chief distinctions that sets us apart from totalitarian regimes." This affirms the right of an American citizen to express his opinion on a subject no matter how offensive it might be or how unpopular it might be with government authorities, state or federal. The judge denied the injunction with these words, "the speaker and the listener, the writer and the reader, and the actor and the observer must be his own watchman for truth, because the founders of our country did not trust any government to separate the truth from the false for the people."

In the April 28, 1972 issue of *Science* there is an article entitled "National Cancer Act: Deciding on People, Policies, and Plans." This act endows the NCI with privileged status and $1.6 billion to spend in the course of the next five years. "Intermingled with lavish and optimistic words of praise for this new enterprise is the often repeated caveat that biomedical research is notoriously an uncertain undertaking, that even the imprimatur of the White House and all that money cannot guarantee success. However, there is some expectation of tangible results." The head of this great endeavor is Frank J. Rauscher, Jr., a scientist who is a well-recognized virologist, who will be directly responsible to the president. There has also been created a National Cancer Panel consisting of one layman and two scientists. Benno C. Schmidt heads the panel. He is managing partner of J.H. Whitney and Company, a New York private venture capital firm that backs developing high-risk businesses with money put up by the partners. The other two members are R. Lee Clark, president of the University of Texas, M. D. Anderson Hospital and Tumor Institute, and Robert A. Good, an immunologist and pediatrician from the University of Minnesota Medical School. F. J. Rauscher is a Ph.D., not an M.D., and his chief contributions have been in the field of animal virology. Several opponents of Rauscher have felt that he is too limited in his concepts, which could be largely confined to carrying on proven procedures, such as Pap smears, mammography for breast cancer, such new techniques for early detection as identification of cancer antigens, and education of both the public and the medical community. Former Director Carl Baker has always argued that research should be geared to solving human cancer problems. The act does enjoin the NCI from spending funds for routine patient care and Baker has contended that cancer control can be equated with patient care. Representative Paul Rogers (D-Fla.) insists that cancer control be written into the legislation, by the president and his aides, the American Cancer Society and Frank Rauscher. The challenge to Rauscher, the panel and the board is one of taking a mass of data reflecting thousands of pieces of research and making some coherent sense of it. Unfortunately much of what is known is erroneous and much that is valuable, constructive and productive has been systematically repressed and interdicted.

Let us hope that freedom will extend to all men in the scientific field who have something to offer to his fellow man that is not surgically obliterative, chemically poisonous, or destructive of body tissues, therapies which can make the healing processes impossible. I am sure that there are many safe and effective modalities in this world that can be sought out for the treatment of the suffering cancer patient. Let us not become an army of obedient, industrious ants completely under the control of an elite medical and political regime where each man's duty is to blindly mouth praises of his oppressors who have the power of life and death over him, dictating whether he should or should not be born, the manner of his life upon the earth, and his method of exit out of this life as a sacrifice to government-controlled science. We must be guaranteed enlightened freedom under God and under our Constitutional rights to govern our own lives and to make our own choices. We serve our country best by enjoying these privileges and rights ourselves and by making certain that they are extended to all of our countrymen whatever their race or creed. We must be true patriots ready to sustain our government and to make sure that it continues by the consent of the governed into paths of law and righteousness.

What Lies
Ahead

A thoughtful friend once said to me, "Everything that we need is right here on this earth. All we must do is to learn how to use it." We have an atavistic longing to return to the Age of Innocence, when the world was a safe, friendly, beautiful place with crystal-clear streams abounding in fish, with meadows and woodlands, fields and pastures offering man food and pleasure for the taking. This was the Garden of Eden, this was Thoreau's Walden Pond. Subconsciously we think that if we could just get back to Mother Nature all would be well with us. When man left the Garden of Eden, he was beset by the woes of the world: starvation, disease, wars, pestilence and various kinds of deprivation. As he crowded into cities he became subject to typhoid, tetanus, cholera, typhus, smallpox, leprosy, tuberculosis, cancer and a host of other ills both physical and psychological expressed by riots and bloodshed at home and by wars in foreign lands, which not only destroy life but also the very soil itself, the source of sustenance for generations to come.

But man has been endowed with superior intelligence and a sense of conscience that sets him apart from the animals. Man has been given dominion over all the earth, for good or for evil. He has been blessed by the efforts of men of good will, by the presence of prophets, teachers and revelators. Man has the power to return the earth to a Garden of Eden, if he will. There have been giants in the world who have lifted up the multitudes. These have been not only men of spiritual attainments but also men of science who have felt strongly the drive to help their fellow man. There is a saying that if one man is raised upward on the shoulders of others and reaches the pinnacle, he can let down a rope and pull thousands up to the same heights.

Since it is men that make nations, then the responsible man must seek to govern and not to corrupt. Great power leads to corruption when any man or group of men has unlimited authority over the minds and bodies of their fellow men. Groups of men must operate as individuals in respect to their identification with each individual who is governed. This is the basis of good government.

The man of science has his responsibilities as well. Every man can learn from reading what is being accomplished by the scientists in his society. Painstaking writers like Patrick McGrady have made every effort to inform the public in simple terms what the progress in curing and treating cancer has been in the past decades. Nutritionists like Adelle Davis have had a great impact on their readers by teaching them the basic facts of nutrition. It takes a brave man like Dr. Roger Williams to point out how lethal a diet of white bread can be, how remiss our standard-makers are in the poor supervision of our foodstuffs. Our infected poultry, our hormone-stimulated cattle, our sheep depilated with chemicals to eliminate the need for shearing, the cruel practice of injecting proteolytic enzymes into living cattle to soften their tissues just prior to slaughter are some of the abuses tolerated by our society.

Our old people are placed in institutions for the aged that are no more than warehouses of the helpless where they are given an impersonal type of care that often is worse than neglect and are fed on devitaminized convenience foods selected chiefly because they are cheap and require a minimal amount of preparation. The profit to the owners of these institutions is phenomenal. There are no real controls as to how much money can be made by the exploitation of the old and the sick. The same thing can be said about our mental institutions. Many of the insane could be released if they were given diets rich in vitamins and high in protein as has been proven with the megavitamin therapy with niacinamide for schizophrenia. Twenty-five to fifty cents is allowed daily to feed each person in some of these places. young people could be trained to farm and provide cheap high-quality food for the old and mentally handicapped.

It seems to me that teaching the young people a purely mechanistic concept of their body is depriving them of some of the most inspirational knowledge that they can ever gain. The human body is an extremely complex mechanism deserving of great respect. Life is a wonder and an amazement. Man, with all his sophistication cannot produce a simple flower or a lowly ant. Albert Schweitzer is an inspiration to us because he revered life in all its forms. Man in many respects is still a savage with primitive, selfish drives. The natural man can be the enemy of the spiritual man. Our children must be taught that the great forces of life like fire and water, sex and hunger, must be channeled and controlled for lasting happiness. Each individual is born with a certain store of emotions and desires that seek fulfillment. Life can become very tawdry if every emotion is cheapened by meaningless repetition. Every animal desire whether for food or sex, if satisfied without forethought, can coarsen and debauch. In brief, the basic verities of life must be passed on to our children.

All of these problems of society are pertinent to the cancer problem. If our children are neglected in childhood, given poor diets high in sugars and low in good nutrients, they may be suffering from a number of nutritional diseases ranging all the way from latent pellagra and hypoglycemia to various border-line diseases such as scurvy. Good health habits are the basis of resistance to disease, including cancer. If the young people practice a life of sexual promiscuity they are exposed not only to venereal disease and various types of latent infections such as cancer, but to the disillusionment that comes from a life without purpose and direction. This attitude toward life leads to the taking of drugs, crime and suicide. We spend untold amounts of money trying to rehabilitate these young people. How much better it would be if each child were planned for, born into a stable home, taught the real values of life, educated to respect himself and others, and to plan for a useful life. We must rise up as a nation and return to the great principles under which our country was founded and which inspired our pioneer forebears to great deeds of accomplishment. The answers are not simplistic. However, the day-by-day guidelines observed by each individual may serve to alleviate some of the problems of our daily living:

Control Your Personal Habits

1. Do not partake of harmful substances that destroy your body such as alcohol, tobacco or drugs. If you are in spiritual accord with your God, your world, and your society you will not need them.

2. Food is an important basis of health. Study books on nutrition. Inform yourself as to what you are eating. Few things can concern you more than what you eat since substances taken into your body become a part of your living cells. If they are good substances they will nourish you. If they are poisonous or destructive, they must be detoxified, destroyed and excreted at considerable cost to the reparative systems of the body.

3. Do not eat anything just because it tastes good. Be sure that you are not tricked into eating poor-quality food because it is sweetened or has a pleasant, piquant or salty taste or because it gives you a temporary lift from its caffeine and high sugar content. Be discriminating. Don't let advertising force you into giving your children sweet, artificially flavored, soft drinks.

4. Learn how to make delicious food and drinks that are healthful and keep them readily available at home and on trips. Do not depend on food processing companies and vendors to determine what you are to eat. At times you are victimized by advertising into eating cheap food with cheap taste appeal. Wake up.

5. Be discriminating. Read all the labels on the food that is offered for sale. Learn to count calories that are present in the sweet syrups and cheap oils that are used in the preparation of the product. How much is good food and how much is camouflage?

6. Check the fresh fruits and vegetables you buy. Are they dyed, covered with an oil to make them look fresh, or sprayed, or show evidence of disease? Do not eat them if they show discoloration or tumorous growth.

7. Keep your young people busy by growing your own garden wherever possible. Teach both boys and girls to cook and prepare healthful meals. These activities provide good family hobbies and will teach children food management which will benefit them and their children for generations to come. Teach them home-maintenance skills.

8. Learn all you can about nutrition. If you become ill, ask yourself what vitamins you are lacking, what essential life substance you may have neglected or what you will need in more abundance during a time of stress or illness. Consult a trusted family physician.

9. Buy your own wheat, rye, oats, flaxseed and other grains. Grind them with a home grinder and prepare your own bread and cereals. Be sure the grains are untreated and uncontaminated.

10. Milk is a good food but remember you are feeding your children all the hormones meant for a young calf. Use milk in moderation and certified if possible. Substitute for milk other high-protein foods such as beans, lentils and whole grains. Read Lappe's *Diet for a Small Planet* as well as the works of such writers as Adelle Davis, Roger T. Williams and Ruth Bennett White. Do not eat chicken or eggs until the poultry industry is cleaned up. Poultry is an excellent source of protein but not in the present diseased state of our fowl.

11. Avoid excessive sweets. Use natural products such as honey, molasses and raw sugars in moderation.

12. Use as many foods as possible uncooked and unprocessed such as nuts, fruits and vegetables.

13. Do not go on fad diets. If overweight, reduce total calories but do not eliminate any essential foods such as whole grains unless supplements are taken.

14. Learn to balance out each day's food requirements as to essential vitamins, raw foods, good quality protein, whole grains, cold pressed fats and oils that contain the essential unsaturated fatty acids, and the total calories needed for each individual member of the family depending on weight, age and activity.

Individual Body Care

1. Cleanliness in your personal habits and in the preparation of foods is a must. Buy a dishwasher. Do not put soiled dishes and raw meats where you are cutting bread or preparing fresh salads.

Keep individual towels and toilet accessories for each person. Use disinfectants on sinks and toilet bowls. Wear clean clothes. Keep your home and bedding clean. Let in the sunshine. Do not clutter up your home with furnishings that are not readily kept clean such as heavy rugs and draperies.

2. Be careful of your personal contacts. Do not have physical relations except with your mate. Promiscuity leads to venereal disease, exposure to cancer and is sinful. Do not take sick people into your home unless absolutely necessary. If you must, provide them with isolation facilities.

3. Keep your body functioning as well as possible by getting sufficient rest and exercise, avoiding undue stress and watching body elimination. Get periodic medical and dental checkups. Eliminate focal infections if they occur. Cultivate your spiritual life. Be useful. Get involved. Help others less fortunate than yourself.

What You Can Demand of Your Government

1. Demand monetary restitution from the government if you are harmed by the use of drugs or biologicals released with government approval such as the Salk and Sabin vaccines. Demand that biological standards be published and made available to the public.

2. Insist that the medical profession keep you informed as to the dangerous side effects of any drugs that are prescribed, even though licensed by government. Many drugs produce iatrogenic disease, that is, disease caused by the drugs themselves. Insist on knowing the prognosis and hazards of treatment with various agents used in cancer if you are a patient. Demand that your prescriptions be labeled with contents, dosage, side effects and antidotes.

3. Demand that all foodstuffs be labeled including the chemical composition of the container in which they are distributed. There are some cans that contain liners that may be carcinogenic. Require that the amounts of sugar, proteins, fats and total calories provided by each ingredient and their percentages be printed on processed food. Beware of empty calories and "fun food" that is junk.

4. Campaign for the investigation of nonlethal medications for the treatment of cancer. Demand statistics.

5. Insist upon cleaning up the poultry industry. All diseased flocks should be destroyed and cancer-free flocks established even if it means relocation of poultry ranches under government subsidy.

6. Try to use other proteins in your menus as a meat substitute such as fish, cheese, whole-grain cereals and nuts.

7. Set up community-sponsored classes in nutrition and public health. Involve the young people in these classes and projects.

8. Monitor all bloods offered at blood banks by darkfield and brightfield examination for the presence of infectious agents. Demand that blood donors have a physical examination before giving blood. Register blood donors.

9. Insist on more rigid controls of sanitation in public eating places.

10. Try to promote isolation and decontamination techniques in hospitals where the acute cancer patient is treated. Do not put a young boy with a tonsillectomy next to an old man with a fresh, draining colostomy for cancer.

11. Insist that your government be more responsible. Where innocent citizens are harassed by a government agency such as the FDA and where they have suffered financial loss due to a lawsuit instigated principally for the purpose of destroying the character of the individual and where the courts have failed to

find cause for such suit, then the citizen should have financial redress through punitive measures against the government agency. Otherwise the taxpayers funds are used to incriminate, harass and destroy innocent people who have no redress under the law.

The cancer problem is just one of the ills of our society. It can be solved if our people will unite and demand investigation of all methods of cancer therapy whether government sponsored or not. We need individuals with consciences and not self-seeking politicians in government. There is enough information available today to provide a real basis for solving this scourge, cancer, the hidden killer.

12. We should support our government by obeying the law and by taking legal corrective measures wherever necessary. We must never forget the sacrifices our forebears made in establishing this country. It is a great privilege to be an American citizen. If our country fails in any way it is because we have failed as individuals. Destructive, nihilistic, and subversive activities should never be condoned. We have a commitment to this wonderful land which has been sanctified by the sacrifical lives of our ancestors. We have a total commitment not only to our country but to our fellow man: to attempt to raise all men from poverty, ignorance, and disease. The conquest of cancer is a primary and outstanding health objective in our country today. The presentation of the truth concerning the present status of cancer treatment in this country is an obligation which the dedicated scientist cannot ignore.

The new approach to the treatment of cancer has taken a wide swing away from the attempt to destroy the cancer cells themselves to a concerted effort to restore the sick host to a state of health by stimulating the immune response so that the diseased condition is overcome by mustering up the inherent natural defense mechanisms of the body. The immunological battle must be won or all else fails. No physician ever healed anyone except by a miracle. It is only the natural healing processes of the body which conquer disease. Hippocrates, the

Father of All Physicians, said, *"Natura Sanat."* Nature heals
The physician is obligated to seek all means to restore health to
the afflicted. Under no circumstances should a patient be
subjected to treatment which is harmful. The motto of the old
Vienna medical school was "Primum non nocere." Above All
Do No Harm.

The basic concept of cancer as an infection which this book
has proposed, can be summarized as follows. It is a natural state
for all living things to be parasitized by various microbes, some
helpful, some harmless and some downright harmful. The
harmful ones usually arouse a state of resistance in the host by
means of various mechanisms such as antibodies, circulating and
fixed white cells, enzymes and numerous other intricate biological processes that seek to restore the body to health. Sometimes the harmful microbes produce substances which prevent
the host from reacting either by elaboration of toxic materials
which destroy the host resistance or by masquerading as a
harmless constituent of the body. Such an invader is the Hidden
Killer, the Progenitor Cryptocides. It can exist in the human
host as an ongoing, underlying chronic infection which, in the
beginning, may be silent but in the end, fulminates into an
overpowering enemy. This subversive third column invader must
be unmasked by recognition of its various forms within the
human body. In the future mass immunization could be developed. Vaccines, antisera, and antitoxins could be produced to
destroy the hidden enemy. Above all, new antiboiotics must be
found. Carcinogens which serve to precipitate the cancerous
disease should be eliminated in so far as possible from the
ecological environment. Methods of controlling this chronic
ongoing, underlying infection must be found. It has been the
purpose of this book to offer means by which some of these
objectives might be fulfilled.

In research it is important to remember never to be intimidated, never to be swayed by public or private opinion, never
to be overawed by big names or great buildings, never to be

overruled by an edict of anyone who has not taken the time to investigate your premises or is incapable of interpreting them due to a lack of desire to learn or an inability to do so. I have tried to work carefully and earnestly taking great pains to arrive at a decision after the best advice and help I could get. As time has passed many of our basic premises have been proven. With the acknowledgment of many of our concepts there is no sense of pride but rather a profound sense of gratitude that we have been permitted to assist our suffering fellow men along the road to freedom from pain and to the fulfillment of a meaningful life cycle upon this earth.

Appendix I

The following was extracted from the American Journal of the Medical Sciences, 220, 638–648, December, 1950, and is reprinted with their permission.

CULTURAL PROPERTIES AND PATHOGENICITY OF CERTAIN MICROORGANISMS OBTAINED FROM VARIOUS PROLIFERATIVE AND NEOPLASTIC DISEASES*

BY VIRGINIA WUERTHELE-CASPE, M.D.; ELEANOR ALEXANDER-JACKSON, PH.D.; JOHN A. ANDERSON, PH.D.; JAMES HILLIER, PH.D.; ROY M. ALLEN, D.SC.; AND LAWRENCE W. SMITH, M.D. From the Bureau of Biological Research (Presbyterian Hospital Branch), Rutgers University.

DEMONSTRATION of the presence of specific microorganisms consistently occurring in tumor cells was first

*Aided by grants from the American Cancer Society, the Damon Runyon Fund, and the Abbott Laboratories of Chicago, Ill. Acknowledgement is made also for the support received from the Presbyterian Hospital, Newark, N. J.

reported by Wuerthele-Caspe in 1947. These organisms exhibited cultural and morphologic features suggesting their possible relationship to the mycobacteria. A symposium reviewing these findings in some detail was published in 1948.[9] Prior to the observation and isolation of these acid-fast organisms from neoplastic tissues of animals and from man, the presence of similar microorganisms in generalized systemic sclerosis (scleroderma), a proliferative collagen disease, had been observed and reported.[10] Following these initial observations, further isolations were made from both blood and tissues of other sclerodermal and cancerous patients. The nature and pathogenicity of these organisms were reported in a preliminary study.[7] The widespread occurrence of these microorganisms in several types of proliferative diseases, and their successful culture outside the body in artificial media, emphasized the importance of a more detailed study of their characteristics. The present paper is an extension and continuation of the previous work.

SCLERODERMA STRAIN. The original cultures isolated on Petragnani and Lowenstein egg media from blood and lesions of patients with scleroderma revealed acid-fast granules of various sizes as well as rod-like forms. Electron-microscope studies suggest that the latter may be linear aggregates of the granular forms. Subcultures of the scleroderma organism taken from the original egg medium grew poorly on Sabouraud's agar. These organisms subsequently were isolated more satisfactorily in an especially devised liquid medium. These scleroderma strains have produced a consistent type of lesion when inoculated into white mice.†

HUMAN MALIGNANT STRAIN. Employing the technique developed in the scleroderma study by Alexander-Jackson and Wuerthele-Caspe,[10] the latter isolated similar microorganisms from the blood of 18 cancer patients, 7 of whom had Hodgkin's disease, by inoculating their blood into chick embryos. Since the chicken has many similar appearing organisms occurring

†A report dealing more fully with the cultural properties and pathogenicity of the scleroderma organism as well as Alexander-Jackson's liquid medium will be presented at a later date.

spontaneously, direct isolations were subsequently made on solid egg media. Unfortunately growth on this artificial medium proved to be feeble and scanty. It was not until Dubos', Alexander-Jackson's, and brain-heart infusion liquid media were used that the organisms could be isolated from human pathologic blood and tissues, and that sufficient growth could be obtained from a similar control series of 17 normal individuals.

SPONTANEOUS ANIMAL TUMOR STRAINS. Concomitant with the study of isolates obtained from human cancer, isolations were also made repeatedly from Rous chicken sarcoma and Sarcoma 180 of the mouse. These cultures likewise reveal a consistent morphology similar to that of the microorganisms found in tissues from cases of human cancer. Although all of these organisms were morphologically similar, yet certain differences, such as rate of growth and size of granules, were found that may aid in their differentiation from one another. The Rous chicken sarcoma cultures were obtained on many media, either from the blood of chickens inoculated with tumor tissue or from the tumor directly. The Rous cultures grew on egg media, blood agar, Dubos' medium, Petroff's medium and other enriched agars. The growth appeared in from 3 to 7 days. Morphologically similar organisms isolated from mouse sarcoma 180 were grown in Dubos' and Alexander-Jackson's liquid media. The granules are characteristically smaller, but otherwise present the same general features as those derived from other groups. More recently, successful isolation of another similar strain of these organisms from a primary lung cancer in a mouse has been accomplished.

MORPHOLOGIC AND CULTURAL CHARACTERISTICS. It has been difficult to classify these organisms on the basis of the usual criteria, that is, morphologic, staining, cultural, and physiologic characteristics. This difficulty is due in large measure to the extremely slow rate and sparsity of growth obtained in the best of culture media. When observed in tissues the organisms are present in both acid-fast and non-acid-fast forms as granules, short rods, and globoid bodies. In culture media minute acid-fast granules predominate in young cultures. As the culture ages, these granules increase in size until they become as large as staphylococci, or even larger, some apparently developing into small acid-fast rod-like forms. Subsequently, the larger granules and rod-like forms appear to pass through the acid-fast state to one which retains the Ziehl-Neelsen fuchsin only when decolorized with ethyl alcohol alone. Ultimately they may lose this acid-fast quality altogether and stain with ordinary dyes. Certain of these rod-like forms contain acid-fast granules while the remaining structures fail to hold the fuchsin stain. This is particularly true of old cultures which contain many of these irregularly staining forms. True branching filaments have not been observed, although unusual forms are often found in old cultures. The granules are gram-positive in character, while the matrix material described below stains poorly.

The variation in size of the acid-fast granules from the lower limits of the light microscope up to a micron or more in diameter has been a matter of great interest. Because of the graduation in size, it was suspected that granules beyond the range of the light microscope might be found. As will be shown, such granules are commonly observed in electron microscope studies. To date we have filtered 10 cultures: 1 sarcoma of human origin, 1 bladder carcinoma, 3 human mammary cancers, as well as 2 cultures from Rous chicken sarcoma, 1 from mouse sarcoma 180 and 1 case of spontaneous breast cancer in a dog. No difficulty was experienced in recovering the cultures from filtrates passing Chamberland L3 and Seitz filters.

These organisms have been grown on the egg media of Petragnani and of Lowenstein, in Dubos' medium, brain heart infusion plus glycerine and various modifications of the latter. A medium devised by Alexander-Jackson for cultivating mycobacteria has given somewhat better growth. Even in blood and serum the growth is slow and never heavy. Because of the characteristic slow growth, cultures of these organisms are grown in tightly stoppered tubes. One of the most typical growth characteristics is the precipitate which forms in cultures in a liquid medium. It resembles a mass of minute granules held together by fine filaments. As growth becomes more obvious the original mass breaks on slight disturbance, forming other small flocculent growths. The supernatant liquid remains clear. Stained slides from young cultures also show this pattern of granules held together by a fine lightly staining network or matrix.[8] This pattern also appears in the electron microscopic studies. On heart-brain agar slants, growth appears after 14 days as very small discrete colonies. In shake cultures of the same media, the growth is confined to the uppermost portion of the tube, but surface colonies are not observed. The organisms appear to be favored by a slightly reduced oxygen tension. An increased carbon dioxide tension did not improve growth in liquid, shake, or agar slant cultures.

The growth characteristics of the organisms isolated directly from the blood of advanced cancer patients in Dubos' liquid albumin medium are most interesting. The organisms appear to be embedded in irregular strands of collagen-like material. The minute acid-fast forms are present as well as aggregates of larger globoid bodies in this matrix. These aggregates strongly resemble groups of mast cells which have disintegrated and released their granules. These forms stain with toluidinblue as do mast cell granules. It seems possible that certain granules which have not infrequently been observed within diseased tissues and which frequently have been called mast cell granules, may be globoidal forms of a microorganism of this type. Similar forms have been reported by Diller,[4] Cuttino,[3] and Grigoraki.[6] The recently published work of Gerlach[5] includes many illustrations corresponding to our own observations.

ELECTRON MICROSCOPIC STUDIES. Many of the smaller bodies were beyond the range of the light microscope and were filtrable on the basis of size alone. Repeated electron microscopic studies were made before and after passage through mice of pure strains isolated from patients with cancer and scleroderma, and from chickens infected with the Rous virus. Preparations were made from both solid and liquid media. The preparation of specimens from the cultures on egg media involved the following procedure: 1) The complete removal of a single colony from the surface without removing any of the medium; 2) the spreading of the colony between microscope slides; 3) the immediate suspension of the organisms in a few drops of distilled water dropped on one of the slides; 4) the evaporation of a small drop of the suspension on a mounted collodion membrane.

The specimens from the cultures in liquid Dubos' medium were prepared in the following manner: 1) Centrifugation of approximately 1 ml. of culture for 5 minutes at 5000 r.p.m. in a small angle centrifuge; 2) resuspending in 1 ml. of distilled water after pipetting off the supernatant liquid; 3) evaporation of a small drop on a mounted collodion membrane; 4) washing the mount after drying with a few drops of distilled water if examination in electron microscope showed the presence of salt.

The growths appeared to consist of 2 distinctly different but intimately related structures. There was a matrix of fine material consisting of small granules 20 mμ to 70 mμ in diameter connected by a mesh of very fine fibers approximately 1 to 2 mμ in diameter. Interspersed in this matrix and physically held in it were more or less spherical and dense granules or globules. These globules had widely varying diameters ranging from 1.5μ to 0.2μ. Their distribution in the matrix was quite characteristic in that individual particles or large closely linked groups were rarely seen. On the other hand, small loose groups of from 2 to 7 globules and "budding" forms consisting of 2 particles of different diameters in close association were very common. The spacing and size distributions of the globules, the presence of "budding" forms, and the lightly staining but unresolved matrix provide the basis for identifying the organism observed with the light microscope in tissue section with those observed in the cultures by the electron microscope.

Pathogenicity Studies. Pathogenicity studies of 4 separate strains of these organisms were undertaken with *a*) 2 isolates made directly from human cancer* patients—the 1st from tissue from a breast cancer; the 2nd from the blood of a patient with advanced sarcoma of the hand; b) an isolate from a Rous chicken sarcoma; and c) an isolate obtained from the 2nd mouse passage of a scleroderma strain derived from a patient's blood. All inoculations were made as a heavy suspension of the culture in liquid media. Twelve mice were inoculated intraperitoneally with 0.2 ml. each of the respective cultures. The 12 control mice received 0.2 ml. of medium. From time to time as the infected mice began to show evidence of disease, they were sacrificed, along with an equal number of controls. Suspensions were made of tissues or blood and then subinoculated into another series. Cultures were routinely made, whenever possible, from all animals sacrificed or dying spontaneously. However, some of the infected animals died and were eaten by their cage mates during the night before cultures could be obtained. A total of 138 mice of unselected strains were used, of which 60 were controls. All 60 controls were examined by post mortem section and culture. Of the infected animals, 35 were similarly cultured and sectioned.

In discussing the pathologic changes induced experimentally in various animals by these organisms, it is well to keep in mind that the problems posed by these studies bear little, if any, relationship to the well established species specificity of such tumors as Rous sarcoma or sarcoma 180 of the mouse. We fully recognize, as do all investigators in the experimental field, that the Rous chicken sarcoma is caused by a virus or filtrable agent and that the tumor cannot be transmitted successfully to other

*Since the breast cancer strain was thought to be attenuated after 18 months of artificial cultures, a freshly isolated culture from the blood of a young boy with advanced sarcoma of the hand was also studied. Both the original breast isolate as well as the one more recently obtained from the sarcoma were inoculated into guinea pigs, both intraperitoneally and subcutaneously. From this experiment, there was little evidence of attenuation of the original breast cancer strain, although the more recently isolated tissue produced more marked proliferative changes in the experimental animals' tissues.

animal species. Similarly, sarcoma 180 must be transplanted into another mouse and ordinarily cannot be induced in any other experimental animal.

The pathologic changes described in this paper are lesions produced *not* by the cells of Rous sarcoma nor by the cells of mouse sarcoma 180, but by any of the several strains of organisms recovered from these and other tumors, including cases of human malignancy. An outstanding feature of interest is that these organisms are apparently not species specific inasmuch as organisms recovered from Rous sarcoma can induce essentially the same response in mice, rats, guinea pigs and rabbits as well as in chickens. Similarly the strain of organisms recovered from mouse sarcoma 180 (or for that matter from any other neoplasm from which this type of organism has been obtained) will produce characteristic lesions when injected experimentally into any of the common laboratory animals.

PATHOLOGIC CHANGES. The lesions may be described in general as pseudo-caseous, rather widely distributed but tending to occur principally in the liver, kidneys, and lungs, although at times involvement of the heart, spleen, adrenal, stomach, and lymph nodes have been noted. In at least 1 instance rather diffuse infiltration of the omental fat was observed.

It is perhaps of significance to note that with each successive animal transplant, the time factor in the development of these lesions tends to be reduced until, in the 3rd or 4th animal passage, it becomes a matter of 10 days to 2 weeks rather than weeks or months. It is also interesting to note that litter mice from infected mothers frequently show identically appearing gross lesions, which as a rule develop only after several weeks. The litters of these mice are usually small in number and stunted.

GROSS PATHOLOGY. A description of any one of these lesions will serve as a pattern for them all, although considerable variation exists in respect to the severity of the reaction, the size and number of the lesions and their distribution. These differences vary, not only with different strains of these organisms but also with individual animals inoculated with the same strain. The typical lesion varies from 2 or 3 mm. up to 8 or 10 mm. in diameter. The majority of these lesions are discrete, but in some instances, particularly in the liver, a number of these small foci coalesce to form a larger conglomerate lesion, occupying perhaps a quarter to a third of the volume of the organ. This is less noticeable in the lungs and kidneys, although even here the same tendency for the lesions to coalesce is observed. No such conglomerate nodules have been noted in the other viscera.

The individual lesion tends to be rather yellowish-gray in color with scattered areas of hemorrhage at times. The lesions are rather nodular in character, and frequently elevated 1 to 2 mm. above the surface of the organ, especially in the liver. In other instances they are buried centrally in the particular organ involved. While these nodular foci are fairly well localized, yet at times they can be seen extending into the surrounding organ and tissues. On section of such a lesion, it appears as a yellow-gray, somewhat firm, elastic caseous area of necrosis, not unlike in some respects that seen in association with tubercle or even miliary gumma formation. As a rule, however, the color is much more yellow than is customarily noted in these 2 other conditions. Neither actual pus formation nor true liquefaction necrosis is found, thus readily differentiating these lesions from any of the ordinary pyogenic infections.

MICROSCOPIC PATHOLOGY. These necrotic foci reveal a basic common pattern, but with marked variation of the picture. The lesion consists of a central area of necrosis made up of masses of organisms occurring almost in colony formation. In hematoxylin and eosin stained preparations, under oil immersion, this necrotic mass can be resolved into a network of eosinophilic staining material in which are embedded tiny globoid bodies tending to stain with the hematoxylin. These coccoid bodies occur sometimes singly, sometimes almost as chains, and at other times in clumps. It also is possible at times to observe coccobacillary forms containing these granules. Toward the periphery of these colony-like masses, the individual organisms can be much more readily distinguished. Here, marked variation in their size and shape is particularly evident with the appearance of short rod-like forms. With Ziehl-Neelsen stained preparations both acidophilic and non-acidophilic forms occur, the acidophilic predominating.*

Surrounding this mass of organisms is a zone of cellular infiltration consisting almost entirely of mononuclear cells of various types, with lymphocytes greatly outnumbering the other types. Large mononuclear phagocytes laden with organisms in both granule and coccobacillary forms are prominent, while plasma cells and other mononuclear cells, difficult if not impossible to identify, are also present in relatively large numbers. Many of these cells undergo degeneration, and free forms of the organism are found in the interstitial spaces. The presence of these organisms likewise appears to stimulate the increase of fibroblasts, and both young and older forms of these cells are regularly found. There is some suggestion that this microbial invasion tends to involve particularly the collagenous tissues. This is particularly seen in the kidney and lung, where the lesions appear principally in the intertubular area and in the alveolar walls, breaking through into the alveoli themselves. This feature is less apparent in the liver, although the fibrous tissue of the portal area is commonly involved.

Comment has been made upon the variations in the basic pattern of this lesion. Nowhere is this more evident than in the animals inoculated with the strains of organisms recovered from a typical Rous sarcoma. The basic lesion still is essentially of a chronic granulomatous nature. The development of no lesion actually resembling the tumor of origin has been observed. Likewise, histologic study of tissues from guinea pigs inoculated

*Careful histologic study of tissues from the 35 experimentally inoculated and 60 control mice mentioned earlier was carried out, sections being stained by routine hematoxylin eosin and Ziehl-Neelsen techniques. All the infected animals showed the presence of the organisms in profusion, while in no instance was it possible to demonstrate them in the control tissues. Similar studies of tissues from guinea pigs inoculated with cultures of this organism gave confirmatory results. Histologic examination of human tumor material taken from over 50 neoplasms of various types and stained with carbol-fuchsin, regularly showed the presence of similar appearing acid-fast and non-acid-fast granules and rods. No organisms could be demonstrated in tissues from normal autopsy cases.

experimentally with the most recent human sarcoma isolate show striking proliferative changes of the fibrous tissue.

Another feature is the not infrequent tendency for necrotic changes to involve blood vessels, both arteries and veins, but particularly the latter. Striking degenerative changes of the connective tissue of the vessel wall are observed, with proliferative changes involving the lining endothelium. In a few instances, where the animal has survived for a sufficient period of time, thrombosis with recanalization of the vessel lumen has occurred. Occasionally, subintimal clumps of mononuclears, indistinguishable from those found in the periphery of the focal lesions, are encountered. As these vessels are usually near the area of caseous necrosis, they may merely represent an extension of the process from vessels passing through the major lesion. At times, however, they have no such apparent relationship and the possibility of the organisms acting directly on the vascular endothelium and vessel wall cannot be excluded.

Summary. 1. A group of morphologically similar microorganisms, varying considerably in size and shape, has been observed in and isolated from various proliferative diseases of man and animals, including scleroderma, human cancer, Rous sarcoma and mouse sarcoma 180.

2. These organisms, which appear primarily as small acid-fast granules in young cultures and which tend to become non-acid-fast in the larger forms present in old cultures, may exhibit a number of types, such as: *a*) minute filterable granules beyond the limits of visibility of the light microscope; *b*) larger granules approximately the size of ordinary cocci, readily seen with the light microscope; *c*) later globoidal forms; *d*) rod-like forms with irregular staining; and *e*) occasionally globoidal forms which appear to undergo polar budding.

3. We have not been able thus far to recover the organism from 17 normal controls nor from patients suffering from any other condition.

4. Cultures inoculated into experimental animals produce a characteristic pseudocaseous lesion. Huge numbers of lymphocytes are called out as part of the response.

5. Final classification of these organisms cannot be made at this time. That they may represent isolated instances of a group of biologically related organisms capable of causing proliferation in the host is not overlooked.

6. Whether these organisms are of primary or secondary significance in the development of malignant disease remains to be established.

Grateful acknowledgement is made to Dr. Royal A. Schaaf, Chief of Staff of the Presbyterian Hospital, Newark, for his invaluable cooperation, to Mr. Paul Little, Lederle Laboratories, for the Rous sarcoma material, to Dr. Sonia Buckley, Sloan-Kettering Institute, for the sarcoma 180 mice, and to Dr. S. A. Goldberg, pathologist, Presbyterian Hospital, Newark, for his kind assistance and advice.

REFERENCES

1. Alexander-Jackson, E.: Ann. N.Y. Acad. Sci., 46, 127, 1945.
2. Idem: Science, 101, 563, 1945.
3. Cuttino, J. T., and McCabe, A. M.: Am. J. Path., 25, 1, 1949.
4. Diller, I. C.: Anat. Rec., 105, 24, 1949.
5. Gerlach, F.: Krebs und obligater Pilzparasitismus, Wien, Urban & Schwartzenberg, 1948.
6. Grigoraki, L.: Edit. Lefrançois, Paris, 1944. From J. Alexander, Colloid Chemistry, Theoretical and Applied, Vol. 7-8, New York, Reinhold. In press.
7. Wuerthele-Caspe, V.: J. Am. Med. Women's Assn., 4, 135, 1949.
8. Idem: J. Med. Soc. New Jersey, 44, 52, 1947.
9. Wuerthele-Caspe, V., Allen, R. M., and Rose, S. J.: Bull. N. Y. Micro. Soc. 2, 1, 1948.
10. Wuerthele-Caspe V., Brodkin, E., and Mermod, C.: J. Med. Soc. New Jersey, 44, 256, 1947.

Appendix II

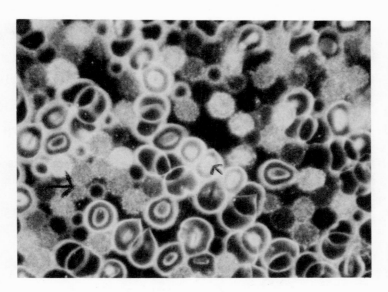

Illus 1. "Target cells" with large inclusion forms. "Spent cells" granular and shrunken. X 750. Sarcoma of the neck.

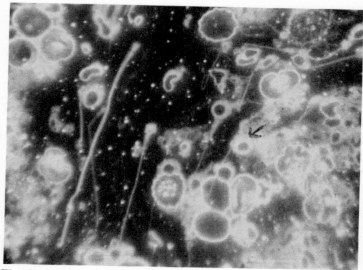

Illus 3. Cyst bodies or mesosomes with vibrating filia at edge. Large motile filaments. Heinz-Ehrlich bodies. × 1,350. Hodgkin's disease of skin.

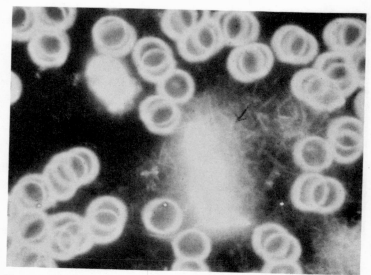

Illus. 5. Shedding of fine spicules from a protoplast. × 750. Carcinoma of the lung.

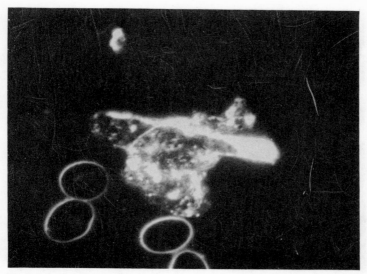

Illus 8. Tubule budding from protoplast. Normal erythrocytes. X 1,350. Hodgkin's disease of the skin.

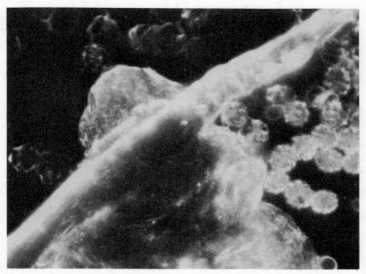

Illus. 9. Development of tubule. X 750. Hodgkin's disease of the skin.

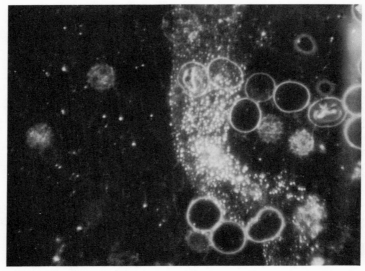

Illus. 10. Breakup of tubule into L-forms. X 750. Sarcoma of neck.

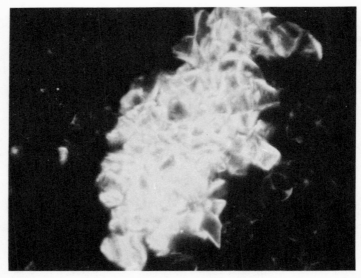

Illus. 11. Protoplast in crystalline form extruding multiple truncated tubules. X 1,350. Sarcoma of the neck.

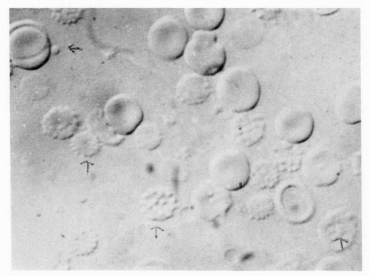

Illus 12. Phase microscope showing Heinz-Ehrlich bodies and "spent cells." X 1,350. Sarcoma of leg.

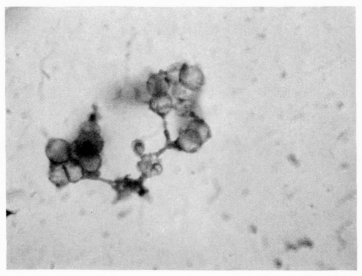

Illus. 15. Interlacing mycelia and budding forms around erythrocytes. X 750. Carcinoma of bowel.

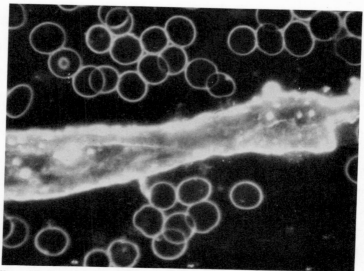

Illus. 19. Large tubular forms with inclusion bodies and extrusion of mesosome. A similar inclusion form is present in an erythrocyte. These smaller inclusion forms might be termed spheroplasts. X 750. Cancer of the lung.

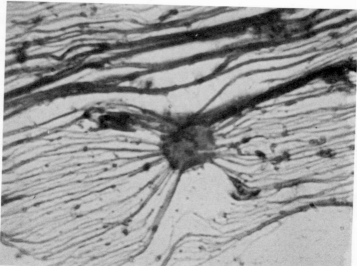

Illus. 20. Mycelial network arising from protoplast. X 1,350. Hodgkin's disease of the skin.

References

Alexander-Jackson, E. 1970. Ultraviolet spectrogramic microscope studies of Rous Sarcoma. Ann. N. Y. Acad. Sci. Vol. 174. Art 2, p. 765.

Baringer, J. R. 1971. Tubular aggregates in endoplasmic reticulum in Herpes Simplex encephalitis. N. E. J. Med. 285(17): 943-945.

Boesch, M. 1960. The Long Search for the Truth about Cancer. G. P. Putnam's Sons, New York.

Cantwell, A. R., and D. W. Kelso. 1971. Acid-fast Bacteria in Scleroderma and Morphea. Arch. Derm. V. 104: 21-25.

Cantwell, A. R., et al. 1968. Acid-fast bacteria as possible cause of scleroderma. Dermatologica. 136: 145-150.

Casey, M. J., Turner, H. C., Huebner, R. J., Sarma, P. S., and Miller, R. J., 1966. Complement fixing antibodies in monkeys bearing tumors induced by Rous sarcoma virus. Nature, 211, 1417-1418.

Cohen, M., R. G. McCandless, G. M. Kalmanson and L. B. Guze. 1968. Core-like Structures in Transitional and Protoplast Forms of Streptococcus faecalis. Ch. 9, p.94-109. Microbial Protoplasts, Spheroplasts, and L-forms. L.B. Guze, Editor, Williams and Wilkins, Baltimore, Md.

Davis, A. Let's Cook It Right. 1970. New American Library, Inc. New York.

Davis, A. Let's Get Well. Harcourt Brace & World, Inc., New York.

Deinhart, F. 1966. Neoplasms induced by Rous sarcoma virus in New World Monkeys. Nature 210, 433.

Delmotte, N. and L. Van Der Meiren. 1953. Recherches bactériologiques et histologiques concernant la Sclérodermie; Dermatologica 107, No. 3 pp. 117-182, Basel, New York.

Diller, I. C. 1962. Growth and morphological variability of three similar strains of intermittently acid-fast organisms isolated from mouse and human malignant tissues. Growth 26: 181-208.

Diller, I. C. and A. J. Donnelly. 1970. Experiments with Mammalian Tumor Isolates. Ann. N.Y. Acad. Sci. 174(2): 655-674.

Diller, I. C., A. J. Donnelly and M. E. Fisher. 1967. Isolation of pleomorphic, acid-fast organisms from several strains of mice. Cancer Res. 27(1): 1402-1408.

Diller, I. C. and W. Diller. 1965. Intracellular acid-fast organisms isolated from malignant tissues. Trans. Amer. Micr. Soc. 84: 138-148.

Fonti, C. J. 1958. Eziopatogenese del Cancro. Amadeo Nicola and C. Milan, Italy.

Guze, L. B. 1968. Editor. Microbial Protoplasts, Spheroplasts, and L-forms. Williams and Wilkins, Baltimore.

Iizuka, H. Naito, A. 1967. Microbial Transformation of Steroids and Alkaloids. University of Tokyo Press, Tokyo, University Park Press, State College, Pennsylvania.

Inglis, B. 1964. The Case for Unorthodox Medicine. G. P. Putman's Sons, New York.

Inoue, S. and M. Singer. 1970. Experiments on a Spontaneously Originated Visceral Tumor in the Newt, Triturus Pyrrhogaster. Ann. N.Y. Acad. Sci. 174(2): 729-764.

Inoue, S., M. Singer and J. Hutchinson. 1965. Causative agent of a spontaneously originated visceral tumor of the Newt Triturus. Nature 205: 408-409.

Kabins, S. A. Interactions Among Antibiotics and Other Drugs, in JAMA The Journal of the American Medical Association, Vol 219, No. 2. January 10, 1972.

Lappé, F. M. 1971. Diet For A Small Planet. A Friends Of The Earth/ Ballantine Book, An Intext Publisher, New York.

L'Esperance, E. 1931. Studies in Hodgkin's disease. Ann. Surg. 93: 162-168.

Levy, B. M., Taylor, A. C., Hampton, S. and Thoma, G. W. 1969. Tumors of the marmoset with Rous Sarcoma Virus; Cancer Res., 29, 2237.

McGrady, P. 1964. The Savage Cell, A Report on Cancer and Cancer Research. Basic Books, Inc. Publishers, New York.

Mazet, G. 1962. Présence d'élèments alcoolo-acid résistants dans les moelles leucémiques et les moelles non-leucémiques. La Semaine des Hôpitaux. (Médicine dans le Monde). 38 e Annee. 1-2: 35.

Livingston, A. M., V. W. C. Livingston, E. Alexander-Jackson, and G. H. Wolters, 1970. Toxic fractions obtained from tumor isolates and related clinical implications. Ann. N. Y. Acad. Sci., 174: 675-689.

Natenberg, M. 1959. The Cancer Blackout, A History of Denied and Suppressed Remedies. Regent House, Chicago.

Necheles, T. F. and Allen D. M. 1971. Heinz Body Anemias. Highlights of Hematology. N.E.J. Med.

Portnoy, J. 1971. Candida Blastospores and Pseudohyphae in Blood Smears. N. E. J. Med. 285 (18): 1010-1011.

Seibert, F. B., F. M. Feldman, R. L. Davis and I. S. Richmond. 1970. Morphological, Biological, and Immunological Studies on Isolates from Tumors and Leukemic Bloods. Ann. N. Y. Acad. Sci. 174(2): 690-728.

Simon, H. J. 1960. Attenuated Infection, The Germ Theory in Contemporary Perspective. J. B. Lippincott Company, Philadelphia.

Smith, P. F. 1971. The Biology of Mycoplasms. Academic Press, New York.

Villequez, E. J. 1955. Le parasitisme latent des cellules du sang chez l'homme, en particulier dans le sang des cancereux. Maloine, Paris, France.

Von Brehmer, W. 1934. Siphonospora polymorpha: Ein neuer Mircroorganismus des Blutes. Med. Welt. 8: 1178-1185.

Waksman, S. A. 1968. Actinomycin, Nature, Formation, and Activities. Interscience Publishers A Division of John Wiley & Sons, New York.

Waksman, S. A. 1950. The Actinomycetales: Their Nature, Occurrence, Activities, and Importance. Chronica Botanica Company.

Watson, J. D. 1968. The Double Helix, A Personal Account of the Discovery of the Structure of DNA, Atheneum, New York.

Williams, R. J. Nutrition Against Disease. Pittman Publishing Corporation, New York.

Wuerthele-Caspe, V. (Livingston). 1955. Neoplastic infections of man and animals. J. Amer. Med. Wom. Ass. 10: 261-265.

Wuerthele-Caspe, V. (Livingston). 1953. A study of a specific microorganism isolated from animal and human cancer. Its identification in tissue. The immunologic aspects both diagnostic and therapeutic. Proc. VIth Int. Cong. Microbiol. Section XVII A. Rome, Italy.

Wuerthele-Caspe, V. (Livingston) and E. Alexander-Jackson. 1965. Mycobacterial forms in myocardial vascular disease. J. Amer. Med. Wom. Ass. 20: 449-452.

Wuerthele-Caspe Livingston, V. E. Alexander-Jackson. 1970. A specific type of organisms cultivated from malignancy: Bacteriology and Proposed Classification. V. 174, Art. 2, 636-654, Ann. N. Y. Acad. Sci.

Wuerthele-Caspe, V. (Livingston), E. Alexander-Jackson, J.A. Anderson, J. Hillier, R. M. Allen and L. W. Smith, 1950. Cultural properties and pathogenicity of certain microorganisms obtained from various proliferative and neoplastic diseases. Am.J. Med. Sci. 220: 638-646.

Wuerthele-Caspe, V. (Livingston), E. Alexander-Jackson, M. Gregory, L. W. Smith, I. C. Diller, and Z. Mankowski, 1956. Intracellular acid-fast microorganisms isolated from two cases of hepatolenticular degeneration. J. Amer. Med. Wom. Ass. 11(4): 120-129.

Wuerthele-Caspe, V. (Livingston) and R. M. Allen, 1943. Microorganisms associated with neoplasms. N. Y. Microscop. Soc. Bull. 2:2-31.

Wuerthele-Caspe, V. (Livingston), E. Brodkin and C. Mermod. 1948. Etiology of scleroderma, a preliminary report. J. Med. Soc. N. J. 44(7):256.

Yamanouchi, K., Fufuda, A., Kobune, F., Uchida, M. and Tsuruhara, T. 1967. Oncogenicity of Schmidt-Ruppin strain of Rous sarcoma virus in cynomologus monkeys. Japan, J.Med. Sci. and Biol. 20, 433-446.

Zilber, L.A., Lapin, B.A., and Adgighy, F.I. 1965. Tumors in monkeys caused by Rous virus. Nature, 205, 123.

Index

Subject Index

Index of Proper Names